Human Factors for Healthcare

Human Factors for Healthcare

A Guide for Nurses and Allied Health Professionals

ALLY ACKBARALLY, RN, DIP H.E NURSING, BSc HONS (NURSING CRITICAL CARE AND PERIOPERATIVE PRACTICE), MSc HONS ADVANCED HEALTH AND PROFESSIONAL PRACTICE, PGCert EDUCATION, FELLOW HEA

Senior Lecturer and Practitioner in Perioperative Care
Health & Life Science, Leicester School of Nursing & Midwifery
De Montfort University
Leicester
England

CATIE PATON, MSc HUMAN FACTORS SCIENCE; PG CERT Ed, FHEA; BA HONS (NURSING); RN

Associate Director of Medical Education, Clinical Skills Consultant
Medical Education
NHS Lanarkshire
Lanarkshire
Scotland

ELSEVIER

Notices

ISBN: 978-0-7020-8487-4

Content Strategist: Andrae Akeh
Content Project Manager: Suthichana Tharmapalan
Design: Ryan Cook
Marketing Manager: Deborah Watkins

Printed in India

Last digit is the print number: 9   8   7   6   5   4   3   2   1

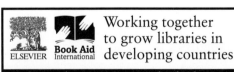

CONTENTS

PREFACE

Welcome to the first edition of *Human Factors for Healthcare: A Guide for Nurses and Allied Health Professionals*. Human factors itself is a well-established science studying the engineering and psychology of human errors in the workplace. Many organisations such as the World Health Organisation, Health and Safety Executives, NHS England, the Chartered Institute for Ergonomics and Human Factors and the Clinical Human Factors Group all attempt to bring human factors to the workplace. However, the concept is only beginning to trickle into the many levels of nursing and allied health professions including the higher and further education institutions. The objective of this book is to guide and support staff to understand and embed human factors in the workplace to deliver the safest practice possible. Our hope is that this book will simplify human factors principles. Therefore the exploration of the concepts will be based on optimising human performance through better understanding of the behaviour of individuals and the team, their interactions with each other and with their environment. This will offer the readers options and ways to minimise and mitigate risk, which consequently will reduce errors and accidents.

CONTRIBUTORS

Anthony Kitchener, Specialist Paramedic, Foundation Degree in Paramedic Science with IHCD Technician and Paramedic Awards, MA in Education, MSc Educational Leadership
Head of Clinical Development
East of England NHS Service NHS Trust
NHS
Peterborough
England

Karon Cormack, BSc Nursing, PGCert Management, PGCert Fronline Leadership & Management, PGCert Human Factors, Improvement Advisor, Certified Coach
Director of Quality
NHS Lanarkshire
West of Scotland University, Open University, De Montfort University, University of Derby, Institute of Healthcare Improvement, Mindful Talent
Glasgow
Scotland

Kay de Vries, PhD, MSc, PGCEA, BSc Hons (Nursing), RN
Professor Older Peoples Health
Health & Life Science, Leicester School of Nursing & Midwifery
De Montfort University
Leicester
England

Lianne McInally, BSc(Hons) Occupational Therapy, MBA Public Services Management
Scottish Improvement Leader, Transformational Coach
Allied Health Professions Senior Manager
Allied Health Professions Services
East Ayrshire Health & Social Care Partnership/NHS Ayrshire & Arran
Kilmarnock
Scotland

Margot Russell, RN, BN, MSc (Medical Anthropology), PgCert TLHE
Director NMAHP Practice Development
NMAHP Practice Development Centre
NHS Lanarkshire
Hamilton
Scotland

Mel Newton, Professional Doctorate, MSc, BSc RN
Special Lecturer
School of Health and Life Sciences
Teesside University
Middlesbrough
England

Ross Thompson, MSc, PgC EAPS, NMC Teacher, AHE Fellow, BN, RN
Lecturer in Adult Nursing
Department of Nursing and Community Health, School of Health & Life Science
Glasgow Caledonian University
Glasgow
Scotland

Zubeir Essat, Dip HE Nursing, LLB, PGCert Education, Fellow HEA
Clinical Educator
Corporate Nursing
University Hospitals of Leicester NHS Trust
Leicester
England

ACKNOWLEDGEMENTS

We would like to thank all the contributing authors who have given their perspectives on the many facets of Human Factors in Healthcare. We are also grateful to the many colleagues who have provided feedback to chapter authors on early drafts. They are not listed but their considered opinion is greatly appreciated and has ensured the formation of this book.

CHAPTER 1

Human Factors in Healthcare

Ally Ackbarally

Introduction

Human factors, or ergonomics, is a well-established field that provides information regarding human and system performance in relation to hazards and safety of organisations, especially in high-risk industries. Unlike healthcare, human factors solutions are well embedded in complex and high risk organisations such as aviation, mining and the military. Human factors encompass the study of human interactions with other people, surroundings, processes, tools and tasks, and the psychology of human errors in all aspects of life such as road traffic accidents, plane crashes, collapse of bridges and medical errors. In other words, finding system solutions for people performance is essential for safe, quality care. Many organisations, such the World Health Organization (WHO), Health and Safety Executives, National Health Service (NHS) England, the Chartered Institution of Human Factors and Ergonomics and the Clinical Human Factors Groups advocate the importance of human factors in healthcare for reducing clinical errors, improving human performance and making the system more resilient. Although there has been extensive research on the topic, it is still not fully implemented in all aspects of healthcare; further, to a certain degree, it is not fully understood by nurses and allied health professionals, including disparities at training level.

This chapter aims at simplifying the understanding of human factors. The concepts will be explored based on optimising human performance, teams, tools, technologies, interactions with the environment and the processes and system as a whole. This will offer the readers options to minimise and mitigate errors and accidents. Furthermore, this chapter provides a general overview of human factors, which will include definitions, a brief history, human factors components and details of some aspects of nontechnical skills. By the end of the chapter, the reader will understand why human factors are important and relevant to nurses, allied health professionals and healthcare systems in general.

WHY DO I NEED TO KNOW ABOUT HUMAN FACTORS?

Most healthcare professionals have heard or read about the Hippocratic Oath 'first do no harm'—including medical practitioners, nurses and allied health professionals (AHPs)—and adhere to the respective code of conduct and ethics (NMC, 2018; HCPC, 2016). Although this is often the first thing taught in any introduction to healthcare ethics, patients are still being harmed every day in hospitals. While some incidences can be considered unavoidable, the vast majority of adverse events that occur in healthcare are avoidable. It is widely accepted that up to 85% of serious incidences in healthcare could be avoided. Some of the most common factors known to cause serious patient incidents—Never Events or other patient related incidences— are results of system errors, communication failures, lack of teamwork, poor environmental design, vital equipment design, blame culture and lack of clinical and organisational leadership.

Very rarely will an incident be related to one specific factor; it is often a combination of factors that bring about the error or the incident. What most incidences have in common is that they are all related to human factors in some way. Therefore, to understand the incidences fully, human factors must be part of any investigation so that the lessons learnt are more meaningful, the system becomes more resilient and the risk of re-occurrence is lowered. In other words, patient safety errors will be at greater risk of occurring if human factors are not part of the solutions and lessons learnt.

Remember your NMC code on preserving patient safety and your responsibility as a registrant.

You need to be aware of, and reduce as far as possible, any potential for harm associated with your practice. To achieve this, you must:

- take measures to reduce as far as possible, the likelihood of mistakes, near misses, harm and the effect of harm if it takes place
- take account of current evidence, knowledge and developments in reducing mistakes and the effect of them and the impact of human factors .and system failures (NMC, 2018, p. 20).

How Are Harm, Patient Safety and Human Factors Linked?

Harm can be a subjective matter in many cases. What is perceived as harm may differ from person to person. For example, a patient may not have been physically harmed—such as with an infection or pressure ulcer—but could have suffered lack of sleep because the ward was very noisy at night and it affected patient health. Thus, perspective is very important, and measurements must include both objective and subjective data. Furthermore, a patient might consider severe pain after surgery as being subjected to harm, despite having a proper pain management plan in place and administering analgesia promptly. The patient can be right even though the healthcare professionals did not necessarily cause harm. This is because the WHO (2019) defines harm as the impairment of structure or function of the body, and any deleterious effect arising from, or associated with, plans or actions taken during the provision of healthcare. It also includes disease, injury, suffering, disability and death, and may comprise physical, psychological or social harm. Conversely, the Agency for Healthcare Research and Quality (AHRQ, 2019) has a more objective stance in defining harm as an act of commission, which is doing something wrong or an act of omission which is failing to carry out the agreed care, i.e. failing to do the correct care that leads to an undesirable outcome for patients. Patient harm in healthcare, such as Never Events, remain constant despite new technology, evidence-based medicine and research (NHS England, 2020). The Health Foundation (2011) links human factors and system failures as being the two most common elements leading to patient harm—the third element being the complexity of care itself. Examples of human factors elements and system failures are staff fatigue, unfamiliar settings, time pressure, failure to acknowledge the prevalence and seriousness of harm and take steps to do something about it, poor communication, assumptions, poor staff to patient ratio, lessons learned from previous incidences not shared adequately and financial difficulties. Therefore, if practitioners are fatigued, stressed and stretched, they will tend to focus on the most essential part of care and may be blinded to holistic care. This is also illustrated by the 12 most common preconditions for errors, known as the Dirty Dozen (Nzelu et al., 2018), which is well known in aviation but also very relevant in healthcare.

The Dirty Dozen includes:

- Lack of communication
- Stress
- Lack of knowledge
- Norms
- Complacency
- Distraction
- Lack of awareness
- Fatigue
- Lack of teamwork
- Lack of resources
- Pressure
- Lack of assertiveness

For example, a patient will get dressings changed or medication on time but will have to wait to speak to someone about concerns—this is when error risks become greater; in other words, the holes in the Swiss cheese slowly align (Fig. 1.1). This may resonate with many practitioners and, sadly, is quite common in practice. It is also important for healthcare practitioners to understand not only what harm is but also the degree or level to which a patient can be harmed (Table 1.1).

Remember Your Patient in Patient Safety

Patient safety, or more importantly the lack thereof, is a global phenomenon recognised by the WHO World Alliance for Patient Safety. The fact remains that one in 10 patients admitted to the healthcare system is harmed, millions of drug errors are made and more than one

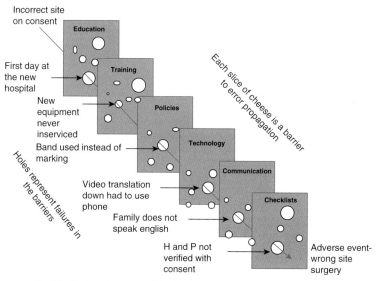

Fig. 1.1   Swiss cheese model of adverse events (Sheesia et al., 2017).

TABLE 1.1 ■ Degree of Harm (NHS Improvement, 2018)

No Harm	Low Harm	Moderate Harm	Severe Harm	Death
A situation where no-harm occurred: either a prevented patient safety incident or a no-harm incident.	Any unexpected or unintended incident that required extra observation or minor treatment and caused minimal harm to one or more persons.	Any unexpected or unintended incident that resulted in further treatment, possible surgical intervention, cancelling of treatment or transfer to another area, and caused short-term harm to one or more persons.	Any unexpected or unintended incident that caused permanent or long-term harm to one or more persons.	Any unexpected or unintended event that caused the death of one or more persons.

million patients die annually of surgical complications globally (WHO, 2019). Although there are many definitions of patient safety in the literature, the NHS England (2019) makes it clear that patient safety is about maximising the things that go right and reducing the things that go wrong for patients and service users. Practitioners, however, know that because of the prevailing organisational culture, investigations tend to focus on what goes wrong and almost never on the system or what people or teams excel at. There should also be serious investigations on near-misses and how practitioners and teams have dealt well with difficult critical situations. This is essentially what Hollnagel et al. (2015) have been advocating regarding the Patient Safety II concept. Otherwise, how are practitioners going to learn the key lessons that make them good at what they do but also how the improvements to make them, the organisation and the system more resilient? Patient safety is a major issue in the United Kingdom given that The Health Foundation (2011) claims that the level of harm in acute hospitals is between 3% and 25%, and approximately 15% in community settings. The National Reporting and Learning System for England continues to report increasing incidences of patient safety (NHS Improvement, 2018). Additionally, Panagioti et al. (2019) concluded that 1 in 20 patients are still exposed to preventable harm; whereas the report 'National State of Patient Safety 2022' by the Imperial College London (Institute of Global Health Innovation, 2022) highlights that systemic safety issues, amongst others, in healthcare have still not been addressed. It is, however, very welcoming that the Care Quality Commission considers patient safety and human factors at the heart of patient care. There is indeed no quality of care without patient safety. Steadily but surely, we are starting to see a paradigm shift in patient safety as professionals and organisations integrate Patient Safety II to Safety I, focusing not only on what goes wrong but also exploring what is being done well and how to sustain and share those best and effective safety practices (Hollnagel et al., 2015). Furthermore, the Systems Engineering Initiative for Patient Safety (SEIPS), part of the PSIRF (Patient Safety Incident Response Framework) (NHS England, 2021) initiative, is a comprehensive tool for healthcare professionals and patient safety investigators to investigate serious incidences (Fig. 1.2). It moves away from linear approaches and takes into consideration the complexity of healthcare and working with people. The SEIPS tool encompasses

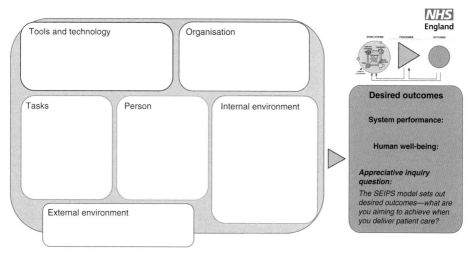

Fig. 1.2 SEIPS tool (NHS England, 2021).

the sociotechnical aspects of the patients' care and journey, including interactions with others, services and processes (Carayon et al., 2020).

A Brief History of Human Factors

Before human factors became common terminology, the study of people at work in the late eighteenth and early nineteenth centuries was widely known as ergonomics, mostly in Europe, which focused mainly on the human interaction with physical work (Parker, 2015). Although the study of ergonomics at the time was not popular in healthcare, attempts were made by Frank and Lillia Gilbreth in the 1900s to reduce errors in surgery by introducing the concept of call backs in the operating room to reduce communication errors (ATM, 2018). The concept developed further, especially with the events of World War I and II and their aftermath, where the aviation and high-risk industries were at the forefront of research and development in the area. Healthcare caught up the 1980s and 1990s, with papers and research highlighting error concepts and human factors contribution, such as those from McIntyre and Popper (1983), Brennan et al. (1991), Gaba et al. (1994), Vincent et al. (2001), the well-known report 'To err is human' (Institute of Medicine, 2000), An Organisation with a Memory (Department of Health, 2000) and now the NHS Patient Safety Strategy (NHS England and NHS Improvement, 2019). However, it was the case reported by Bromiley (2015) that truly highlighted the role of human factors in the health service in the UK. In 2005, his wife went for what is considered a routine ENT surgery, and sadly died a few days later due to a complication with intubation ('can't intubate, can't ventilate') in the anaesthesia room. Being an airline pilot, Martin ensured that the incident was investigated, and the lessons learned from that event highlighted the importance of human error and nontechnical skills—essentially human factors in healthcare.

What Are Human Factors?

Think about how many times you have done something wrong because of bad designs; for example, have you ever walked into a door thinking it was a push door but it turned out to be a pull door, or how many times do you rush out of the house, stressed and in a hurry to beat the morning traffic, only to realise you forgot the car keys inside the house or worse, have locked yourself out? In healthcare, certain common lapses such as taking the controlled drug keys to the canteen may not have a severe implication on patient safety but administering the wrong medication (Fig. 1.3) to the wrong patient or operating on the wrong patient will end up in severe harm, if not death.

These unfortunate common events in healthcare are more than likely caused by human error or factors that caused the person(s) or team(s) to act incorrectly or deviate from the correct course. Healthcare practitioners working in all areas of healthcare normally do an incredible job day in day out; they are excellent at prioritising tasks, making sense of complex clinical or critical situations that arise and constantly having to move from one task to another for 10- or 12-hour shifts. This means that, sometimes, practitioners will miss something important, misunderstand communications, assume things (assumption bias) or even cut corners knowingly or unknowingly. Practitioners are not only physically tired but mentally and cognitively exhausted. Therefore, many are under enormous pressure due to workload and stress while juggling organisational targets along with patient safety and staff well-being. It is very easy to understand why errors occur and why another Mid-Staffordshire disaster is not a fiction (Martin et al., 2023).

When the errors, incidences or harm to patients or staff occur, key questions one must ask are:
- Do the investigations also include use of human factors tools and principles?
- Are nontechnical skills studied?
- Are the incidences simulated and re-enacted?
- Are lessons shared to seek answers and solutions?

More often than not the investigations tend to focus on the sharp end of people and do not include the 'blunt end' or a system approach which will provide understanding rather than blaming. These are just a few examples of the vast science that is human factors and most of these events occur in healthcare.

Defining Human Factors

In certain areas of hospitals, such as in anaesthesia and surgery or among professionals working in clinical simulations, it seems like you cannot have a conversation on patient safety without hearing about human factors. However, is the term well understood amongst

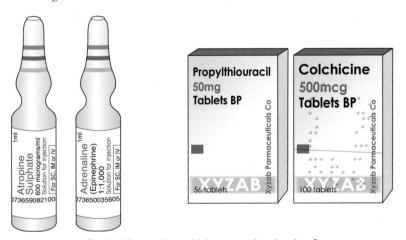

Fig. 1.3   How easily could the wrong drug be given?

healthcare professionals, and is it embedded in practice where it matters the most? Why are some areas more receptive to implement human factors than others? These are some of the questions practitioners should be asking and reflecting upon to build a learning and patient safety culture.

As a term, 'human factors' is sometimes interchangeably used with ergonomics or together. This can cause confusion in the mind of practitioners and renders the concept vague or too semantic for mass buy-ins. There is, however, a ratified, recognised, international definition for human factors as a 'scientific discipline concerned with the understanding of interactions among humans and other elements of a system, and the profession that applies theory, principles, data, and methods to design in order to optimise human well-being and overall system performance' (International Ergonomics Association, 2000). In simpler words, human factors is a discipline that provides an understanding of what affects performances and behaviours in the workplace, how we work cognitively and physically and how to design the work environment and systems to maximise safety and reduce errors. Ergonomists will be very articulate with those terms, but this can still feel overwhelming when looking at it from a novice perspective. Healthcare practitioners need to feel more at home with the definition and concept, so that it can be assimilated in practice and healthcare education more readily. Ives and Hillier (2015) managed to make the concept more usable in healthcare by advocating its benefits to improve 'human performance, optimise well-being, improve both staff and patient safety and experience and improve the overall system performance', especially if human factors is applied to the organisation as a whole. Furthermore, the National Quality Board set up a concordat following the aftermath of The Mid Staffordshire NHS Foundation Trust Public Inquiry (2013), regrouping major national organisations which agreed that human factors can play a crucial role in improving patient safety, reducing errors and improving the culture of safety in organisations as a whole. The National Quality Board adopted the definition of human factors in healthcare by Catchpole (2010): 'enhancing clinical performance through an understanding of the effects of teamwork, tasks, equipment, workspace, culture and organisation on human behaviour and abilities and application of that knowledge in clinical settings'.

What are the Elements of Human Factors?

Human factors comprise a broad-based science encompassing disciplines such as applied psychology (clinical and experimental), anthropometrics, cognitive sciences, engineering, systems of organisations and safety engineering (Table 1.2). This is because people have different capabilities, abilities, coping mechanisms perceptions and personalities; interact differently with their environment; and are affected by events differently—therefore, they will face different challenges. These are only a few examples, but the key point here is that human factors aim to understand all these elements and contributions to errors in the workplace and to provide solutions so that these errors can be minimised or avoided. However, the integration of human factors in the workplace or the organisation does not happen overnight and can be complex, especially in healthcare. Normally there is not just one simple answer to improve the system or how to prepare practitioners to work differently, which can be met with resistance and barriers. One must simply consider how long it took to implement the safety checklist in operating theatres that are currently accepted as mandatory practice. Nevertheless, adopting an approach to consider human factor in the workplace should make it easier for healthcare practitioners to do the right thing and more difficult to do the wrong thing. Thus, understanding and integrating human factors in practice will ultimately lead to safer care, better outcomes, more resilient staff and a reduction in human errors.

TABLE 1.2 ■ AMT Handbook, 2018 (Chapter 14)

Clinical Psychology	Psychology applied for the purpose of understanding, preventing, and relieving psychological distress or dysfunction and to promote subjective well-being and personal development. For example, helping practitioners deal with stress, improve coping mechanisms or dealing better with negative feedback.
Experimental Psychology	The study of a variety of basic behavioural processes such as learning, perception, human performance, motivation, memory, language, thinking, communication, physiological behaviours and problem solving.
Anthropometrics	The study of the dimensions and abilities of the human body. Understanding this science is key to safety, including staff safety in relation to assistance in surgery, patient moving, handling and prone positioning.
Cognitive Science	The interdisciplinary scientific study of minds as information processors.
Safety Engineering	A field of study ensuring that life-critical systems perform as intended even when the component fails. In healthcare, it is not only about equipment but also about how the safety system or processes cope to preserve safety when a key operator makes a mistake.
Organisational Psychology	The study of relations between people and work. It includes organisational structure and change, job satisfaction, training and personnel development.
Industrial Psychology	An organised approach to the study of work, including working standards, and conditions, environment and statistical analyses of safety performance.

Human Error

To understand human factors, the practitioner must also understand the concept of human error. Most practitioners studying patient safety have heard of the phrase 'to err is human' (Institute of Medicine, 2000), meaning that people can and will make mistakes, mostly unintentionally; however, intentional errors or deviations exist. The Health and Safety Executives (2020) define human error as an unintentional action or decision, possibly an error of commission or omission, whereas intentional errors or violations are deliberate actions. Fig. 1.4 shows an adapted human error classification encompassing nontechnical skills and intentional and unintentional failures.

The starting point for practitioners is to understand the core principles of human error, including human error classifications. Is the error intentional or unintentional? It is essential not to overlook the latent conditions of an institution which can lead to both intentional and unintentional errors. For example, fatigue can play a part in slips and lapses, but a workplace tolerating defiant practitioners can also very likely lead to intentional errors. It is not always as clear-cut as it seems—sometimes a practitioner can deviate from the norms to save a patient's life or deviate from the policy to speed up a procedure; thus, the intention is crucial here. This introduces the concepts of 'work as imagined' versus 'work as done', and brings into question policies, guidelines and standard operating procedures. Are they well written, and can they be followed in practice? Are they fit for the purpose? These need to be considered as a systematic approach to policy, guidelines and standard operating procedures. Will it support staff and make it easier to do the right thing, thus avoiding blame culture? Additionally, it is also important to understand that human error does not happen in a vacuum; it normally occurs when conditions such as poor nontechnical skills and lack of supervision, teamwork and/or leadership are aligned. Recognising other clues such as mental overload, stress or bystander apathy is pivotal to support colleagues.

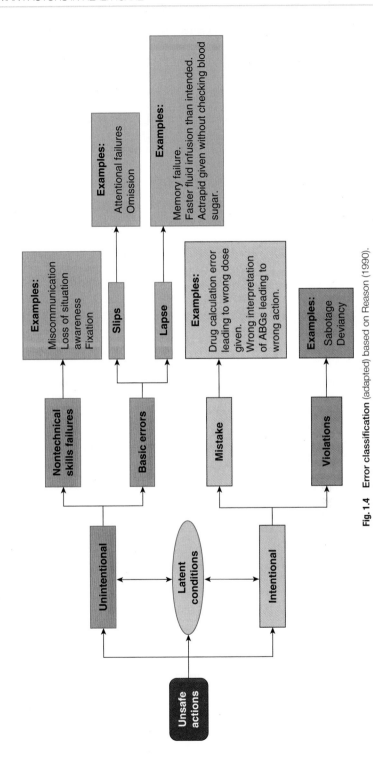

Fig. 1.4 Error classification (adapted) based on Reason (1990).

Acknowledgement of these issues will minimise the risk of further complications and is crucial in establishing trust in teamwork.

It is unfortunate that at times individuals are blamed for incidences or adverse events mostly owing to linear approaches to investigations that only use root cause analysis tools (Peerally et al., 2017). Usually, frontline staff such as nurses, operating department practitioners (ODPs), pharmacists and medical practitioners feel the brunt of those investigations and are sometimes labelled as unsafe, careless, forgetful, negligent or downright reckless. How many times have hospitals reviewed and updated their safety policies for the same error or mistake that happens again? However, it can be true that someone is reckless or forgetful, but how do we know they truly are? How many times did they forget to do something crucial? It could be advocated that staff who trigger regular incidences should be supported further as they may have an accident-prone personality trait and may be prone to making errors. This does not mean that they are to be blamed for errors but supported and coached to be more efficient at their roles. Hogan (2016) mentioned that the most common accident prone personalities are namely:

- Defiant
- Panicky
- Irritable
- Distractible
- Reckless
- Arrogant

In contrast, the system approach to human error does not blame the individual. Errors are not necessarily seen as a personal or individual failure, but rather a consequence of the organisation or system shortcomings, and countermeasures are based on improving the system to minimise individual errors (Reason, 2000). A prime example of this philosophy in action is the Swiss cheese model of systems and accidents (Reason, 2000), wherein safeguards and defences such as policies, guidelines, supervision, mentoring or peer review and assessing are put in place to minimise errors. If considered comprehensively, the Swiss cheese model can highlight active and latent failures such as systems shortcomings, poor designs, poorly written policies or guidelines, low staffing, time pressure, stress or blame culture. Improvement to patient safety can only be made if both active and latent failure are addressed. The Swiss cheese model, however, is only as good as its users; it has its limitations but can be useful. Although the model is not often used in the methodological sense, one of the ways it can help with safety is to simulate or test the prevailing system for identifying weaknesses and loopholes, which represent potential failures that can be 'gated' (Seshia et al., 2017) and safeguarded as shown in Fig. 1.1.

Nontechnical Skills

What affects one's performance during driving a car, piloting an aeroplane or performing a clinical task in a hospital is multifaceted, especially as explained by human factors. It could include how individuals or teams interact with everything around them, and the effects from the nontechnical skills of the person or the team at that particular time. Much research and investigation into patient adverse events have highlighted failures of nontechnical skills as a major factor leading to incidences. Nontechnical skills can be defined as cognitive, social and personal skills that complement and enhance technical abilities or skills for safe and effective task performance (Flin et al., 2008). The full concept will be explored in the nontechnical skills chapter (Chapter 5).

Nontechnical skills are crucial, because failure to demonstrate one of them can lead to patient harm. Some examples of nontechnical skills are situation awareness, communication, leadership, task management, managing stress, decision-making, coping with fatigue, complacency or coping with pressure.

Furthermore, nontechnical skills are not only a theoretical concept but are also tangible as highlighted in the Bromiley incidence (Bromiley, 2015). They are an element of human ability that can be improved, coached and assessed with validated tools. Have you been assessed as a practitioner? How do you know you possess good nontechnical skills especially in stressful or critical situations? Do you know your strengths or limitations when communicating in stressful situations? Can you lead or will you be fixated on a specific task? These are the questions practitioners and employers need to consider when conducting training needs analyses to improve individual and team performance to face any scenarios. What affects your performance at work (Fig. 1.2)? Think of all the possible barriers as well as solutions.

Exercises

Review the following case studies and reflect on how you would analyse the incidences without any input from human factors, and then including human factors by comparing and contrasting the results and how lessons can be learned (Case Studies 1.1 and 1.2).

CASE STUDY 1.1 **Local Anaesthetic Local Line Flush (CORESS, 2011)**

I undertook open insertion of a double lumen Hickman line in a paediatric patient undergoing chemotherapy for osteosarcoma. The case proceeded normally. The line was tunnelled from chest wall to cervical region, using the blunt tunnelling device in the kit, and inserted into the internal jugular vein. The line tip position in the right atrium was confirmed by image intensifier. The venotomy was closed with 6.0 Prolene and both lumens of the Hickman line, back-bleeding having been demonstrated satisfactorily, were flushed with heparinised saline. Just prior to closing, I realised that I had inadvertently tunnelled the line through the pectoralis major muscle, rather than superficial to it. Concerned that this might cause pain or early occlusion, I removed the line and re-sited it superficial to the muscle. The radiographer was called back to the theatre to re-confirm line tip position. After checking luminal back-bleeds again, I asked the scrub nurse for the heparinised saline and flushed both luer locks and line lumens. At this point the scrub nurse realised that she had given me a syringe containing bupivicaine instead of Hepsal flush. Both syringes had been contained in the same kidney dish, appropriately labelled with circumferential grey and white stickers around the syringes.

The incident described above could have happened in any care setting, at any time and by anyone involved in drug administration. Do not consider the incident as an isolated event.

In relation to human factors: What steps were missed in applying the correct procedure here? What do you think led to the wrong medication being administered?
- Tips
- Distraction
- Fixation
- Assumption
- Communication
- Guideline/procedure not followed
- Teamwork
- Organisational failure

Now categorise the failures:
- Active failure
- Latent failure
- Nontechnical skills
- System

CASE STUDY 1.2	**Drug Error in Intensive Care**

Nurse 1

'It was 2 a.m. and my patient was due paracetamol 1 g P.O. administered through the nasogastric tube because he was intubated. I could not find the purple oral syringe that I would normally use and instead used a luer lock syringe to aspirate the paracetamol before administration. Just before I administered the paracetamol, my charge nurse at the next bed called me to give her a hand with a turn in a pressing tone. I didn't feel I could ask her to wait and instead told my colleague at the next bed to administer the drug so I could go help my charge nurse. I told her it was already checked and ready to be administered. I don't know why I did that, but I was tired and I felt I could tell her to do my task as she was my friend'.

Nurse 2

'I was very happy to help and since the drug was already checked and ready, it should have been quick as I know the patient as well. The drug was in a luer lock syringe and I assumed it was an intravenous administration and I gave it through the central line. I could not see any bubbles or small particles in the syringe as the main lights were off to allow the patients who were not sedated to sleep. I was a bit tired as well. Upon completion of the administration the patient suffered a heart attack'.

Although here the mistake was clear and obvious, procedure was not followed as in relations to human factors. Analyse what went wrong here in relation to human error and nontechnical skills.

- Tips
- Power gradient
- Confirmation bias
- Inattentional blindness
- Change blindness
- Assumption
- Tiredness
- Environmental factors
- Communication
- Assertiveness

Now categorise the failures:

- Active failure
- Latent failure
- Nontechnical skills
- System

HOW CAN HUMAN FACTORS HELP?

Human factors and ergonomics are already embedded in certain areas of practice in healthcare; they make a real difference to patient safety (Fig. 1.5). For example, user interfaces such as monitors, syringe drivers, ventilators or anaesthetic machines are being designed to be more user-friendly and help operators in terms of different alarm sound recognition, warning lights or easy to troubleshoot steps. Routine or daily equipment that healthcare professionals use are also being redesigned to make them safer. For examples, oral liquid medications are given in oral syringes that cannot be connected to intravenous (IV) devices and epidural connections and vice versa, or spinal or epidural syringes cannot be accidentally connected to IV or arterial devices. On an individual level, nontechnical assessment

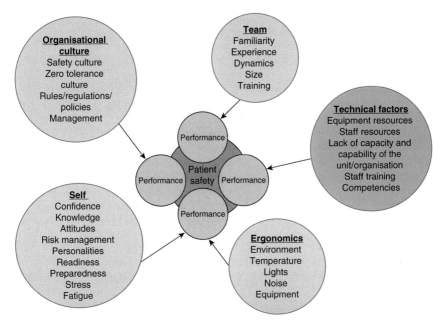

Fig. 1.5 Technical and nontechnical skills affecting performance.

tools such as the NOTTS (non -technical skills tool for surgeons) for surgeons (University of Aberdeen, 2012), the ANTS (anaesthetists' nontechnical skills) for anaesthetists (Flin et al., 2010) and the SPLINTS (scrub practitioners' list of intraoperative nontechnical skills) (University of Aberdeen, 2010) for theatre practitioners (nurses and ODPs) exist to support those individuals to improve their specific nontechnical skills and develop their own individual safety nets—thereby making them safer practitioners especially during critical events. However, should there not be a universal nontechnical assessment tool for nurses working in medical and surgical wards, mental health nurses, midwives and paramedics? There are still many potential areas where human factors can help. The operating theatre safety checklist introduced by the WHO to improve teamwork and minimise errors is rooted in human factors, especially research from the aviation industry. How do we know the team we work with works well together or can perform well in a critical event? Has a simulation been conducted or has the team been assessed objectively? How many times do you get to practice adverse events that may happen in areas where you work and are given the chance to improve your weaknesses, such as assertiveness, excel at what you are good at or build team resilience? Tools such as the OTAS (observational teamwork assessment for surgery) (Hull et al., 2011) and the Team Performance Observation Tool (TeamSTEPPS 2.0) (AHRQ, 2014) can be used for assessment, feedback and team support for further improvement and how to work well together as a unit. Gradient assertiveness tools can also improve communication especially in stressful and critical situations for practitioners who may find it hard to communicate in those situations.

Human factors tools or models exist to support investigations of serious patient safety incidences and shed light on very important lessons, reasons and contributing factors behind the errors that happened in the first place. The tools are multidimensional and will guide the investigators on approaches and line of enquiry. Some of the common human factor tools used in healthcare investigations not mentioned in this chapter are:

- Healthcare Failure Mode and Effect Analysis (HFMEA) (De Rosier et al., 2002)
- Software-Hardware-Environment-Liveware-central Liveware (SHELL) (Hawkins and Orlady, 1993)
- Human Factors Analysis and Classification System (HFACS) (Scott et al., 1997)
- Systems, human interactions, environment, equipment, personal (SHEEP) (Rosenorn-Lanng and Michelle, 2013).

Furthermore, it is also crucial to understand how work is done, what the exact steps are and what needs to happen for the outcome to be accomplished. Understanding how work is done will bridge the gap in how work is imagined; this will make practice safer. The system will be more resilient as policies, guidelines and procedures are updated in line with how work is done. This activity can be illustrated using the Hierarchical Task Analysis tool (Iflaifel et al., 2021). Through the PSIRF initiative, NHS England (2021) advocates the use of further tools such as Link Analysis and Walkthrough Analysis to support understanding of the tasks performed and to reduce the gap between work as imagined and work as performed.

System Thinking

It is inconceivable that healthcare will continue to use a myopic approach to incident investigations. In healthcare, especially in the United Kingdom, the NHS is one of the most complex organisations in the world with more than one million individuals in the system with different personalities, strengths, weaknesses, workplace culture, norms and values. This combination makes it even more complex. So why do we reduce investigations to simplification and use simple linear tools such as Root Cause Analysis or Fishbone analysis? The PSIRF (NHS England, 2021) initiative is a breath of fresh air when it comes to system thinking and patient safety improvement. Investigations can now be more comprehensive and address the shortcomings that may otherwise be missed or ignored. The SEIPS tool can encompass system thinking as it encourages using wider perspectives in contrast to other linear tools. Fig. 1.6 presents an example of a blood transfusion incident investigation recorded and summarised on a SEIPS tool. Other benefits of system thinking are that it considers staff well-being and safety and attempts to address the cultural nuances and barriers in the workplace (Kelly et al., 2023). For more insight into system thinking and what it means to healthcare, please see video at https://www.youtube.com/watch?v=5oYV3Dqe0A8.

Conclusion

It is important to realise that although it is difficult to completely eliminate errors and incidences in healthcare, it is crucial that they are reported as human factors are part of the investigations. Healthcare staff are incredibly resilient and given the opportunity and support, improvement can escalate drastically. Nurses and allied health professionals on the frontline can be assessed and trained to improve their overall nontechnical skills, so that they can interpret situations leading to errors, rectify course and have contingencies in place to avoid the errors that may arise. Improving patient safety is multifactorial (Fig. 1.2) and every single factor, in addition to culture and resilience, should be taken into account for meaningful improvement. System thinking and system factors will need to be part of the way we think and do things because it is not only important that we understand how errors and incidences occur but also how we can do the right things and get them right.

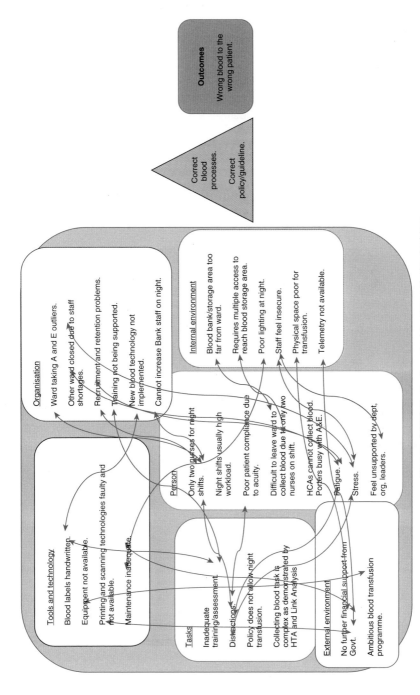

Fig. 1.6 SEIPS illustration of a blood transfusion incident.

Key Points

- Errors and patient safety incidences can be very expensive for organisations and devastating for healthcare staff, patients and families. NHS claims are approximately £2.69 bn.
- Human factors, leadership and communication are frequently identified as root causes for sentinel events.
- You have to learn from adverse events (CIEHF, 2018).
- Patient safety and human factors can be integrated in healthcare and healthcare curriculum (Academy of Medical Royal Colleges in collaboration with Health Education England, NHS England and NHS Improvement, 2020; Carthey, 2013; Patient Safety Movement, 2020; WHO, 2011).
- Embed human factors in practice (Kelly et al. 2023).

References

Academy of Medical Royal Colleges in collaboration with Health Education England, NHS England and NHS Improvement, 2020. National Patient Safety Syllabus 1.0. Training for All NHS Staff.

Agency for Healthcare Research and Quality, 2014. Team Performance Observation Tool. https://www.ahrq.gov/teamstepps/instructor/reference/tmpot.html.

Agency for Healthcare Research and Quality (AHRQ), 2019. Adverse Events, Near Misses, and Errors. https://psnet.ahrq.gov/primer/adverse-events-near-misses-and-errors.

Aviation Maintenance Technician Handbook, 2018. Aviation Maintenance Technician Handbook – General. U.S. Department of Transport and Federal Aviation Authority.

Brennan, T.A., Leape, L.L., Laird, N.M., Hebert, L., Localio, A.R., Lawthers, A.G., et al., 1991. Incidence of adverse events and negligence in hospitalized patients. Results of the Harvard Medical Practice Study I. N. Eng. J. Med. 324 (6), 370–376.

Bromiley, M., 2015. The husband's story: from tragedy to learning and action. BMJ Qual. Saf. 24 (7), 425–427.

Carayon, P., Wooldridge, A., Hoonakker, P., Hundt, A.S., Kelly, M.M., 2020. SEIPS 3.0: human-centered design of the patient journey for patient safety. Appl. Ergon. 84:103033.

Carthey, 2013. Implementing Human Factors in Healthcare. 'Taking Further Steps'. 'How to' guide: Volume 2. Clinical Human Factors Group. www.chfg.org.

Catchpole, K., 2010. Cited in Department of Health Human Factors Reference Group Interim Report. National Quality Board. March 2012. https://www.england.nhs.uk/ourwork/part-rel/nqb/ag-min/.

CIEHF, 2018. White Paper. Human Factors for Health & Social Care. https://ergonomics.org.uk/resource/human-factors-in-health-and-social-care.html.

CORESS, 2011. CORESS Feedback (Ref 110). https://www.coress.org.uk.

Department of Health, 2000. An Organisation with a Memory: Learning from Adverse Events in the NHS. The Stationery Office, London.

DeRosier, J., Stalhandske, E., Bagian, J.P., Nudell, T., 2002. Using health care failure mode and effect analysis™: the VA National Center for Patient Safety's prospective risk analysis system. Jt. Comm. J. Qual. Improv. 28 (5), 248–267.

Dupont, G., 1997. The Dirty Dozen errors in aviation maintenance. In: Proceedings of 11th Federal Aviation Administration Meeting on Human Factors Issues in Aircraft Maintenance and Inspection: Human Error in Aviation Maintenance. Federal Aviation Administration/Office of Aviation Medicine, Washington, D.C., pp. 45–49.

Flin, R., O'Connor, P., Crichton, M., 2008. Safety at the Sharp End: A Guide to Non-Technical Skills. Aldershot, Ashgate.

Flin, R., Patey, R., Glavin, R., Maran, N., 2010. Anaesthetists' non-technical skills. Br. J. Anaesth 105 (1), 38–44.

Gaba, D.M., Fish, K.J., Howard, S.K., 1994. Crisis Management in Anesthesiology. Churchill Livingstone, New York.

Gordon, R., Flin, R., Mearns, K., 2005. Designing and evaluating a human factors investigation tool (HFIT) for accident analysis. Saf. Sci. 43 (3), 147–171.

Hawkins, F.H., Orlady, H.W., 1993. Human Factors in Flight. Avebury Technical, Aldershot.

Health Care Professions Council (HCPC) Standards of Conduct, 2016. https://www.hcpc-uk.org/standards/standards-of-conduct-performance-and-ethics/.

Health and Safety Executives, 2020. Human Factors/Ergonomics – Managing Human Failures – HSE. https://www.hse.gov.uk/humanfactors/topics/humanfail.htm.

Hogan, R., 2016. The accident-prone personality. People & Strategy 39 (1), 20–24.

Hollnagel, E., Wears, R.L., Braithwaite, J., 2015. In: Hollnagel, E., Wears, R.L., Braithwaite, J. (Eds.), From Safety-I to Safety-II: A White Paper. National Library of Congress, Washington, D.C.

Hull, L., Arora, S., Kassab, E., Kneebone, R., Sevdalis, N., 2011. Observational teamwork assessment for surgery: content validation and tool refinement. J. Am. Coll. Surg. 212 (2), 234–243.

Iflaifel, M.H., Lim, R., Crowley, C., Ryan, K., Greco, F., 2021. Detailed analysis of 'work as imagined' in the use of intravenous insulin infusions in a hospital: a hierarchical task analysis. BMJ Open 11 (3): e041848.

Institute of Global Health Innovation, 2022. The National State of Patient Safety 2022. What We Know about Avoidable Harm in England. Imperial College London, London.

Institute of Medicine (US), 2000. Committee on quality of health care in America. In: Kohn, L.T., Corrigan, J.M., Donaldson, M.S. (Eds.), To Err Is Human: Building a Safer Health System. National Academies Press (US), Washington D.C.

International Ergonomics Association, 2000. Human Factors/Ergonomics (HF/E). https://iea.cc/what-is-ergonomics/.

Ives, C., Hillier, S., 2015. Human factors in healthcare common terms, clinical human factors Group. Working with Clinical Professionals and Managers to Make Healthcare Safer. https://www.chfg.org.

Joint Commission Online, 2015. A complimentary publication of the joint commission. Most frequently identified root causes for Sentinel Events January 1–December Patient Safety 31, 2014. 2,378 total https://www.jointcommission.org/.

Kelly, F.E., Frerk, C., Bailey, C.R., Cook, T.M., Ferguson, K., Flin, R., et al., 2023. Implementing human factors in anaesthesia: guidance for clinicians, departments and hospitals: guidelines from the Difficult Airway Society and the Association of Anaesthetists. Anaesthesia 78 (4), 458–478.

Martin, G., Standford, S., Dixon-Woods, M.A., 2023. A decade after Francis: is the NHS safer and more open? BMJ 380, 513.

McIntyre, N., Popper, K., 1983. The clinical attitude in medicine: the need for a new ethics. Br. Med. J. 287 (6409), 1919–1923.

National Health Service England, 2021. Patient Safety Incident Response Framework. https://www.england.nhs.uk/patient-safety/incident-response-framework/.

National Health Service England, 2020. Provisional Publication of Never Events Reported as Occurring between 1 April and 30 September 2020. https://www.england.nhs.uk/wp-content/uploads/2020/11/Provisional-publication-NE-1-April-30-September-2020-.pdf.

National Health Service England, 2019. The NHS Patient Safety Strategy. Safer Culture, Safer Systems, Safer Patients. NHS Improvement and NHS England.

National Health Service Improvement, 2018a. Developing a Patient Safety Strategy for the NHS. Proposal for Consultation. NHS Improvement, London.

National Health Service Improvement, 2018b. NRLS National Patient Safety Incident Reports: Commentary. NHS Improvement, London.

NHS England and NHS Improvement, 2019. The NHS Patient Safety Strategy. Safer Culture, Safer Systems, Safer Patients. https://www.england.nhs.uk/wp-content/uploads/2020/08/190708_Patient_Safety_Strategy_for_website_v4.pdf.

Nursing & Midwifery Council, 2018. https://www.nmc.org.uk/standards/code/.

Nzelu, O., Chandraharan, E., Pereira, S., 2018. Human factors: the Dirty Dozen in CTG misinterpretation. Glob. J. Reprod. Med. 6 (2):555683.

O'Daniel, M., Rosenstein, A.H., 2008. Professional communication and team collaboration. In: Hughes, R.G. (Ed.), Patient Safety and Quality: An Evidence-Based Handbook for Nurses. Agency for Healthcare Research and Quality (US), Rockville. chapter 33.

Panagioti, M., Khan, K., Keers, R.N., Abuzour, A., Phipps, D., Kontopantelis, E., et al., 2019. Prevalence, severity, and nature of preventable patient harm across medical care settings: systematic review and meta-analysis. BMJ 366, I4185.

Parker, S.H., 2015. Human factors science: brief history and application to healthcare. Curr. Probl. Pediatr. Adolesc. Health Care 45 (12), 390–394.

Patient Safety Movement, 2020. Actionable Patient Safety Solutions (APSS) #17: Patient Safety Curriculum.

Peerally, M.F., Carr, S., Waring, J., Dixon-Woods, M., 2017. The problem with root cause analysis. BMJ Qual. Saf. 26 (5), 417–422.

Reason, J., 1990. Human Error. Cambridge University Press, Boston.

Reason, J., 2000. Human error: Models and management. BMJ 320 (7237), 768–770.

Rosenorn-Lanng, D., Michell, V., 2013. The SHEEP Model: Applying Near Miss Analysis. https://www.researchgate.net/publication/297364889.

Scott, A., Shappell, S.A., Wiegmann, D.A., 1997. A human error approach to accident investigation: the taxonomy of unsafe operations. Int. J. Aviat. Psychol. 7 (4), 269–291.

Shesia, S.S., Bryan Young, G., Makhinson, M., Smith, P.A., Stobart, K., Croskerry, P., 2017. Gating the holes in the Swiss cheese (part I): expanding professor Reason's model for patient safety. J. Eval. Clin. Pract. 24 (1), 187–197.

The Health Foundation, 2011. Evidence Scan: Levels of Harm. www.health.org.uk/levelsofharm/.

The Mid Staffordshire NHS Foundation Trust Public Inquiry, 2013. Report of the Mid Staffordshire NHS Foundation Trust Public Inquiry. The Stationery Office, London.

University of Aberdeen, 2010. Scrub Practitioners' List of Intraoperative Non-Technical Skills (SPLINTS). Structuring observation, rating and feedback of scrub practitioners' behaviours in the operating theatre. Printed by UniPrint, University of Aberdeen.

University of Aberdeen, 2012. The Non-Technical Skills for Surgeons (NOTSS) System Handbook v1.2. Structuring observation, rating and feedback of surgeons' behaviours in the operating theatre. University of Aberdeen, Royal College of Surgeon of Edinburgh and NHS Education for Scotland. Printed by UniPrint, University of Aberdeen.

Vincent, C., Neale, G., Woloshynowych, M., 2001. Adverse events in British hospitals: preliminary retrospective record review. BMJ 322 (7285), 517–519.

WHO, 2011. Patient Safety Curriculum Guide Multi-Professional Edition. Patient Safety. A World Alliance for Safer Care. https://www.who.int/publications-detail-redirect/9789241501958.

WHO, 2019. Patient Safety. Key Facts. https://www.who.int/news-room/fact-sheets/detail/patient-safety.

CHAPTER 2

Human Error

Ross Thompson

Ross Thompson

CHAPTER AIMS

1. Introduce the concept of human error
2. Explore what errors in human factors are and are not
3. Examine a serious incident where human factors played an intrinsic role
4. Understand the pressures which can lead to errors
5. Develop strategies that help to avoid errors
6. Discuss what you should do when an error occurs

Introduction

The field of human factors, sometimes referred to as ergonomics (Wilson, 2014), has long sought to understand how human beings interact with the system or environment in which they work. It is considered that by examining these interactions we can understand how to improve performance (Parker, 2015). Naturally, in high-risk safety conscious industries such as healthcare, human factors research has focused on reducing risk, mitigating errors and improving safety. Russ et al. (2012) state that the roles of human factors in healthcare are to support the work healthcare providers undertake and crucially, to facilitate the highest and safest standards of patient care.

The drive to examine the causes of errors is present in almost all safety driven industries—two prime examples of which are healthcare and aviation. A common approach in human factors research is to look at an industry or workplace as a system (Wilson, 2014). By analysing the different tasks which take place within the system, we can start to understand how it works and where we could improve its running. When we think about healthcare as a system, there are innumerable tasks that take place daily, such as performing a surgical operation, dispensing a medication or delivering a terminal diagnosis. The way these tasks are performed and the results they generate vary depending on the setting, time of day and resources available, among many other factors. There are many healthcare professionals for example doctors, nurses, physiotherapists, radiographers and clinical support workers, and their interactions with the healthcare system differ. At the centre of the system, there is the patient who is extremely important, but also variable and dynamic. Human factors research aims to examine this system, identify where we can optimise performance and potential error risks and introduce measures to mitigate those risks (Parker, 2015; Scanlon and Karsh, 2010).

Professor Sheona MacLeod: Director of Education and Training NHS England

Patient safety has to be everyone's priority. Until every healthcare worker knows that 1, they should speak up when they see a risk, 2 they will be respected for doing so, whatever grade they are, and 3 they will not be blamed if they admit when they make a mistake, we will still have a number of significant safety issues occurring in our NHS. So encourage all team members to be open about concerns, treat their concerns seriously and explain your thinking if your expertise makes you think there is no risk, and support colleagues when they make mistakes. Realising you made an error feels awful, it feels hard to admit it, but supportive leaders and colleagues enable healthcare staff to learn to do so.

Therefore, encourage all team members to be open about concerns, treat their concerns seriously and explain your thinking if your expertise makes you think there is no risk and support colleagues when they make mistakes. Realising you made an error feels awful and hard to admit but supportive leaders and colleagues enable healthcare staff to learn to do this.

The value of human factors in healthcare is well established. The World Health Organization (WHO, 2011) acknowledges human factors repeatedly in its influential curriculum for patient safety. The WHO argues that human factors failures play a role in almost all healthcare errors and assert the importance of not only prioritising improvements but also educating healthcare providers from the beginning of their training (Tingle, 2011; WHO, 2011). In the United Kingdom, the importance of human factors was highlighted by the findings of the Francis report (Mid Staffordshire NHS Foundation Trust Public Inquiry, 2013). The Francis report was published after a public enquiry into the serious failings at the Mid Staffordshire NHS Foundation Trust. Although the report does not explicitly mention the term 'human factors', it identifies a number of human factors failures which led to errors and negatively affected patient safety. The report summary identified a system that did not place the safety of patients at its core but rather values which supported its own proliferation (Mid Staffordshire NHS Foundation Trust Public Inquiry, 2013). It proposed that a dangerous culture had developed, wherein concerns were not taken sufficiently seriously, that the organisation did not make enough effort to measure the effects the system had on patients and a failure to tackle problems which negatively affected both patients and staff (Mid Staffordshire NHS Foundation Trust Public Inquiry, 2013). In response to this report, the NHS in England published a concordat (National Quality Board, 2013), with the intent on demonstrating they understood the importance of human factors in patient and staff safety and asserted their commitment to integrate human factors principles into the health service. This concordat acknowledges the importance of adopting the principles of human factors service-wide, helping to support a culture wherein the safety of the patient and wellbeing of staff at its heart. It also recognised the importance of analysing systems from a human factors perspective, and identifying safety risks, learning and changes that can be made to make the system safer (National Quality Board, 2013).

What Are Errors in Human Factors and Who Is Responsible?

It is helpful to first consider what errors in human factors are and are not. Russ et al. (2013) state that there is some dissonance in academic literature as to what constitutes an error in human factors. They assert that there is a misconception that human factors errors are focused on an individual person's failings rather than the failing of a system or process wherin error is allowed to occur (Russ et al., 2013). It is believed that this misrepresentation of human factors is unhelpful when trying to integrate them into modern healthcare and counterproductive to improving patient safety (Russ et al., 2012, Russ et al., 2013). When we look at errors in human factors in healthcare, we seek to understand how we as human beings interact with the health system and how we can make this as efficient as possible.

Roth et al. (2017) point out that nurses, like all healthcare workers, are human—and therefore bound to make mistakes. In the course of a shift, we can go through any number of physical, psychological or social changes which can affect the way we perform our work. We could be tired after a long run of shifts, have had to skip a lunch break because of a sick patient or have had an argument with a co-worker which is playing on our minds. All these and many more factors can affect the way we go about our work, meaning we may interact differently with the system. This may be the point where we make a mistake, an upsetting prospect for any healthcare provider. The role of human factors research is not to identify the point at which to blame someone for an error, it is to help develop a system that can compensate for the variability of the humans who interact with it and mitigate the risk that can therefore occur. Human factors are not just a personal venture. Carayon et al. (2014) acknowledge the complexity of healthcare systems and the role human factors play in them. They go on to assert that to effectively integrate positive human factors in healthcare, all levels, from individuals to national organisations, need to be considered (Carayon et al, 2014). Interventions which only focus on the personal level are usually limited and rarely have significant effects (Carayon et al., 2014). For example, identifying that nurses on shift were recurrently tired which led to errors being made. A limited approach would be to tell the nurses to get more sleep and provide a seminar on mindfulness and sleep hygiene. A more comprehensive approach may consider, in addition to this approach, how to address the problem at a leadership and organisational level. This could mean supporting staff to balance shifts with other responsibilities such as caring for a relative, considering shift patterns and whether staff rotas were not providing enough recovery time. On an organisational level, policy could be created so that staff had to complete a questionnaire or similar before shifts to assess their fatigue level. This system is used in a number of safety critical settings, including retrieval medicine, as a way of mitigating the errors associated with fatigue. These are only a few examples to help to demonstrate the comprehensive nature of human factors.

James McLean: Deputy Chief Nurse, Incident and Operations Director Health Education England

Systems can and do fail, often adversely affecting patient safety. It is important to recognise, report and learn from these episodes and ensure we reduce the risks of reoccurrence. Any event of this nature can be quite disruptive and disturbing for any individual involved, inclusive of the patient, carer and/or family. Direct support, debriefing and recovery actions with peers and leaders is paramount to develop a work programme that will truly close the loop and enable improvements to be enacted and adopted. Honesty and integrity take courage, and standing up for improvement does too. Education is key to the delivery of quality improvement and embedding best practices to reduce risk. Patient safety is the responsibility of everyone.

Errors in Human Factors Which Led to Disasters

Errors resulting from human factors have been linked to a number of high-profile incidents including the space shuttle Challenger disaster, the crashing of a Nimrod aircraft in Afghanistan in 2006 and the Chernobyl nuclear disaster (Haddon-Cave, 2009; International Atomic Energy Agency, 1992; Presidential Commission on the Space Shuttle Challenger Accident, 1986). These incidents had significant human costs as well as financial, environmental and socio-political effects which are still felt today. You may be asking how these disastrous events relate to a medication error or drug miscalculation by one nurse on a ward. The mistakes made in the Challenger case and in the control room of reactor four in Chernobyl have and do happen in wards, cockpits and offices every day. These tragic incidents differ only in setting and scale from those human factors errors which routinely occur but go unreported or unnoticed. The errors which lead to big disasters can also lead to smaller mistakes; thus, by examining these errors we can identify strategies to mitigate them and reduce their chances of reoccurrence. We are going to explore one of these incidents in Case Study 2.1 and identify some of the key human factors failures.

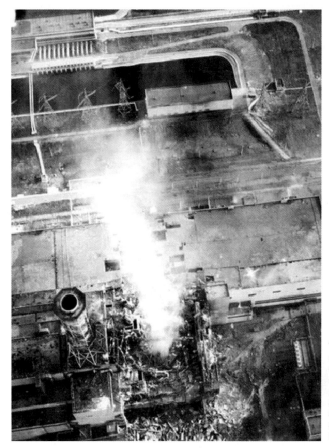

This image of the Chernobyl site was taken 7 days after the explosion. The fire can be seen still raging below, sending radioactive dust up into the atmosphere which would spread all over the surrounding areas as well as large parts of northern Europe.

CASE STUDY 2.1: Chernobyl Nuclear Disaster, 1986

There are few incidents in our recent history which demonstrate the potential for tragedy when human factors failures occur better than the Chernobyl nuclear disaster. This incident occurred in a nuclear facility on 26 April, 1986, in the former Union of Soviet Socialist Republics (modern-day Ukraine) (Plokhy, 2018). In their historical account of the disaster, Plokhy (2018) describes how a test of one of the reactors' safety procedures had been planned to take place on the previous shift, requiring the reactor's energy output be brought down steadily to a safe range which would have been lower than the norm in order to complete the test. Unfortunately, after the power level reduction of the reactor had begun, the government office responsible for energy output in the region delayed the permission to lower energy output further to meet the demand for energy for approximately 10 hours. This delay had a number of effects on the physics of the reactor—the details of which we will not be discussing—and the human factors which affected the reactors.

The original test was planned to take place on a shift made up of controllers with more experience, partly to ensure safety but also to ensure overall smooth running and success. This appears to have been a primary concern for the plant management who were keen to meet targets, increase output, reduce delays for repairs and safety inspections and generally impress. However, by delaying the test to a later shift, the controllers involved were less experienced and ill-prepared to carry out the complicated, highly pressurised test. Due to the nature of the nuclear reactor, its power could not easily be increased and decreased quickly in a safe way. This meant that when the safety test was postponed, the reactor was kept running at a lower level for a longer time than anticipated by the design engineers. This led to a chain of reactions; when the safety test was undertaken, the reactor was not ready and the energy output dropped to extremely low levels, effectively stalling.

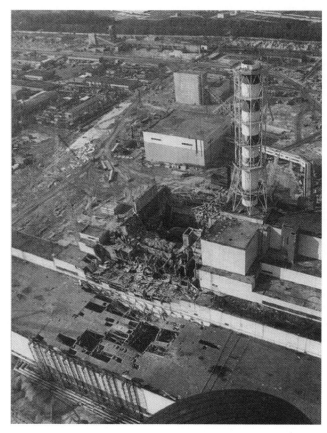

This image shows the destroyed reactor hall of the Chernobyl power station after the disaster. The roof is completely destroyed exposing the walls and ruptured reactor below.
The roof was partially destroyed by a 2000 tonne plate of metal and concrete which was blown up through it by the initial blast, landing back on top of the reactor on its edge.

This would have been an embarrassing blunder for the controllers and reputationally damaging for the plant managers who would have missed out on the successful test completion target. Contrary to safe operating procedure, the lead controller on the shift ordered that control rods, which help to safely control the rate of the nuclear reaction within the reactor, similar to brakes on a car, be removed in large numbers. The intention of this was to increase the power output of the reactor to quickly allow the safety test to be run as planned. Other controllers on the shift knew this was dangerous but either felt unable to challenge the lead controller or were not listened to. The lead controller on that shift was known for his authoritarian, hostile and unapproachable personality. By removing control rods, the reactor did begin to increase power output, although still too low to safely begin the test. Despite this, the chief controller ordered the safety test to begin. Shortly afterwards there were two extremely large and powerful explosions from the reactor. This caused the immediate loss of life of several engineers in the hall which housed the reactor, who had no idea the test was even taking place, and the release of vast amounts of deadly radiation. This incident led to a large number of deaths directly linked to the event and many thousands from the cloud of radiation which spread across the surrounding area and eventually large parts of northern Europe. The legacy of the Chernobyl nuclear disaster includes one thousand square miles of contaminated, uninhabitable land, life-limiting health conditions and contribution to the collapse of the Soviet Union. There were a number of key errors in human factors which played a significant role in the Chernobyl disaster that we in healthcare can learn from.

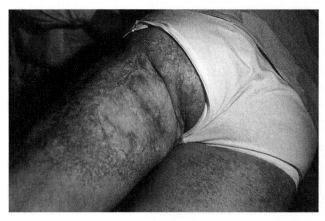

This image shows the scaring left by radiation burns after five years on the thigh and buttock of a Chernobyl firefighter. As firefighters were the first to respond to the explosion and had little knowledge or experience of dealing with radioactive material, many picked up highly contaminated material or sat on contaminated ground.

TARGET FOCUS

The first error in the Chernobyl disaster was prioritising meeting targets rather than safety. The focus on the desired outcome of the activity rather than the process meant that safety was less of a concern. It is common in healthcare to have to work towards certain targets. These can be official targets such as the 4-hour target, wherein a patient is assessed, discharged or admitted in UK emergency departments within 4 hours of presentation. These targets can also be unofficial—for example, having all your patients up and washed for the day shift coming on. It is important to say that not all targets are bad or will lead to errors. In fact, when used appropriately, healthcare targets can remind us to complete some tasks, emphasise the importance of tasks, and help prioritise. There are two significant pitfalls in the use of targets which can lead to them becoming counterproductive. The first is when everything becomes a target. A checklist may seem like an appropriate measure to take when an error has occurred. However, when everything is a target, the items lose their significance and it becomes harder to know what should be prioritised. Creating targets is just one tool in our toolbox and will not work in every instance. The second pitfall is when targets are so inflexible that they have to be completed even when their completion could lead to poorer outcomes—for example, when a patient in an emergency department is discharged before adequate assessment or treatment in order to not breach the 4-hour target. Any rule needs to be suitably flexible to work safely in the real world.

EXPERIENCE AND PREPAREDNESS

The second human factors failure to consider from the Chernobyl disaster was the lack of consideration given to the resources available on that night and experience of those undertaking the test. The team who undertook the test were unprepared, given little warning of the task they were undertaking and included a number of less experienced controllers (Plokhy, 2018). In healthcare, it is common for teams to have similar issues. A team of nurses on a shift can comprise a mixture of nurses more experienced, who have not long joined the unit, those newly qualified and bank nurses. This team will likely change every shift, meaning the team dynamic is never consistent and nurses cannot always know what they can expect from or what they can rely on from their colleagues. The team on a given shift may have to complete complex tasks with little warning or preparation such as helping to place a chest drain, attend an important meeting or react to an acutely deteriorating patient. These are challenging situations and they require effective management and leadership to be addressed. Efforts should be made to achieve a safe mix of skills in a team, so that there is enough knowledge and experience available in the shift that will also allow more junior staff to obtain experience and learn from their more experienced colleagues in a supportive environment. This could be as simple as considering skill mix when organising staff shifts, but can also include planning the personal development of staff and their education.

LEADERSHIP

The final factor we will discuss is the team leadership during the Chernobyl disaster. The lead controller was an experienced team member; however, he was also authoritative, confrontational and had little time for questions. During the test, he repeatedly snapped at those in his team and shouted at them to hurry up (Plokhy, 2018). This leadership style alienated those he was leading and meant that they did not feel comfortable asking questions or expressing concerns. In healthcare, we have many leaders including hospital managers, ward managers, more experienced nurses, operating department practitioners and associate physicians unofficially leading more junior professionals working alongside them. The people in these positions have a great degree of influence over those in their team, and their decisions can have serious consequences (Arnold and Boggs, 2020). Good leaders need to be able to display a range of desirable qualities, manage their own stress besides that of their team and navigate the most effective leadership style for the situation. All of these are skills which require training, support and experience to achieve consistently. It is important to also stress that the position of a leader does not put them beyond questioning. As we saw with the Chernobyl team, a leader who does not listen to different views or whose team feels that they cannot question their direction will cause errors. A flattened hierarchy accommodates a leader who can successfully steer and direct their team while also considering their contributions, knowledge and experience.

Liz Simpson: Clinical Nurse Educator

If you are part of a visiting team (e.g. clinical emergency team), remember you are there to help. Do not judge! You have no idea what the staff's day has been like before you arrived. Remain calm, polite, professional and above all else, approachable. If you do not, the people you are there to help may be too intimidated to provide you with key information. When you need help from someone, always make eye contact with them, introduce yourself, ask them their name, then ask them to do what you need them to do and to let you know the outcome. How long does it take to say 'Hi, I'm Liz. What's your name? Can you take the vital signs for me please and let me know what they are Jamie? Thanks.' These few seconds saves so much time in the long run and enhance patient safety.

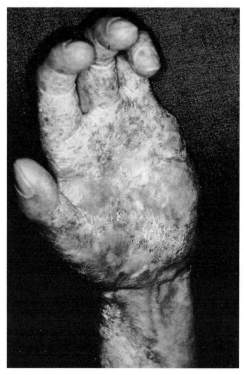

This image shows the hand of a Chernobyl survivor fifteen years after the explosion.
The scarring caused by radiation burns, cutaneous radiation syndrome, is still very visible and extensive.
It can also be seen that a digit has been lost as a result of the burns and that they have caused contraction of some other digits.

Although the legacy of any disaster is unenviable, lessons can be learned. The aftermath and investigations of the Chernobyl disaster led to human factors being taken more seriously. It also led to the term 'safety culture' being coined, expressing the intention to place safety at the forefront of an organisation's collective goals. Both the space shuttle Challenger and the Nimrod reviews also made recommendations to improve safety and human factors which went on to have significant effects on their respective organisations. For example, the UK Ministry of Defence (2014) published the Manual of Air Safety, an influential document which outlined a number of safety practices and standards, and took steps to introduce a more safety-focused culture in the Royal Air Force.

Adverse incidents, whether they be large scale disasters or small errors, are emotive and difficult when they occur; however, when they do, there is a responsibility to examine their causes and learn from their mistakes.

What Pressures or Stresses Can Lead to Errors?

It is useful when examining errors in human factors, to consider the pressures and stresses which can cause them. Working in healthcare, pressure is a constant factor in our work (Hall et al., 2016; Institute of Medicine (US), 2000). They can be time pressures, such as a district nurse getting through their cases in time to change a syringe driver before it finishes or having to prepare a patient for an urgent surgical procedure. They can be technical, for example a nurse practitioner assessing an injured ankle or correctly dressing a wound using sterile technique. They can also be personal, for instance having had an argument at home before shift or taking on extra shifts because of money worries. These are only a few examples of the innumerable pressures which we as healthcare providers experience every day that can affect the way we carry out our duties. It is also important to consider more positive pressures. Motivation to complete a task can be internal, such as satisfaction completing a job, or external, such as receiving praise. This can be a powerful tool for improving performance and is considered a positive pressure.

Dr Kerr Brogan: Consultant Opthalmic Surgeon

When overloaded, multitasking leads to error. No matter how busy you are, take a deep breath and focus on the task at hand. When this is complete, breathe and move onto the next job.

Pressure and stresses are inescapable parts of both our professional and personal lives; however, they are not always a bad thing. An experiment conducted on animals by Yerkes and Dodson (1908) found that in some more complex tasks, the application of a stressful stimulus could positively affect performance initially; however, as the level of stimulus increased, a peak in performance was reached followed by an overall decline in performance. This work has gone on to be influential in the field of behavioural sciences, known as the Inverted U Theory. Although there are criticisms of the Yerkes and Dodson (1908) theory (Diamond, 2005; Sandi, 2013), there are a number of supporting academic sources (Diamond, 2005; Hearns, 2019; Mendl, 1999) as well as corroborating anecdotal and observational evidence. Hearns (2019) proposes a model where pressure can both aid and hinder our performance in healthcare settings, based on the work of Yerkes and Dodson (1908). Hearns (2019) states that there are three levels of performance which correspond to the level of pressure we are put under (Fig. 2.1) (Kelly et al., 2023).

The first level is Disengagement, where there is little or no pressure on us to complete a task. An example of this could be filling in a form at work which you feel has little importance. As you do not feel there is much importance in or pressure on you to complete the task there is less incentive to complete or make time for the task. This is a dangerous level of engagement as although our perception is that this task is not engaging or perhaps less important it could still have consequences if it is completed incorrectly. Engaging people in these tasks is a real challenge and it is not always easy making people see the value in tasks which may appear tedious and without obvious reward. One of the key roles of human factors in this instance would be to find ways to engage staff and have them invest in the task process. Part of the mandatory revalidation process nurses must undertake in the United Kingdom requires them to complete several reflective accounts about their practice. This incentivises nurses to reflect on their professional practice as well as on how they are developing and learning, because without it they would not be allowed to practice.

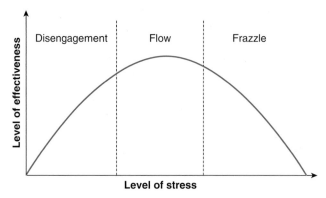

Fig. 2.1   Three levels of performance corresponding to pressure level; adapted from Hearns (2019).

The second level of performance Hearns (2019) describes is called Flow. This occurs when the level of pressure is just right; we feel the importance of the task we are completing, invested in the outcome and engaged in the process. When we are in the flow level, there are still stresses and pressures, but we are equipped to deal with them because they are at an optimum level, not too little to have us disengage and not too many to leave us overwhelmed. An example of this would be when you are working and kept busy with tasks and requests but have the time to complete each effectively and feel confident in your skills to complete them. From a human factors perspective, this is the sweet spot and requires a lot of thought and good planning to consistently achieve.

The final level of performance Hearns (2019) describes is called Frazzle. This occurs when the level of pressure or stress is so great that we are overwhelmed, unable to safely and effectively complete our task. In a frazzled state, we are stunned by all the stimuli being thrown at us and cannot think clearly enough to consistently work at our optimum, be that fast, safe and accurate. These stimuli can take many forms—for example, the quantity and complexity of tasks you are asked to complete, the limited amount of time to complete them and the environment you are in when trying to undertake them. Although we can complete tasks in this state, we struggle more and more, even to the point of being paralysed with indecision. Hearns (2019) asserts that, at this level, we can experience a fight or flight response to the situations we find ourselves in. Experiencing this type of threat response is itself very stressful, can affect the decisions we make and lead us to become defensive or aggressive to those around us. All of these factors can negatively affect task completion and contribute to errors being made.

The Hearns (2019) model explains the importance of pressure on how we work, that pressure needs to be manageable and we need to control it in order to get the best performance. In any task we undertake, there are numerous pressures we can experience. Some of these are associated with the task itself and some with the persons, group or organisation carrying it out. These pressures have been categorised as intrinsic and extrinsic pressures (Hearns, 2019) (Fig. 2.2).

Intrinsic pressures are pressures that are inherent to the task itself. These pressures will be the same for everyone completing the task, although different people will experience them differently. These intrinsic pressures are a result of the attributes of the task such as its complexity, length of time needed to complete it, its importance, amount of knowledge needed to complete the task and the risk associated with it. The more intrinsic pressures that are associated with a given task, the harder we may find it to complete the task. For example, consider a drug round where you are dispensing medications. This is a complex task as you have a large number of patients who all have numerous different medications to take. The drug round takes a significant amount of time to do

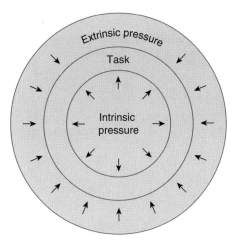

Fig. 2.2 Intrinsic and extrinsic pressures; adapted from Hearns (2019).

safely—you need to focus on the task and cannot safely help to do other things. You know it is very important to dispense the medications as it forms a crucial part of your patients' treatment. You need to have a lot of knowledge about the different medications and their doses, side effects and interactions with other drugs in order to complete the round safely. There is also a risk that if you make a mistake during the drug round, perhaps giving the wrong drug or the wrong dose, you could cause serious harm to a patient.

In a perfect world, we would be able to observe these intrinsic pressures, identify the weaknesses or risks which are created and make changes to address them. Unfortunately, we also have to consider the arguably more dynamic and difficult to address extrinsic pressures. Extrinsic pressures are the pressures which are not directly attributed to the task itself but can still affect its completion. These pressures are changeable, dynamic and more dependent on the circumstances in which we complete a task. Some examples of these are the task setting, how you feel when you are undertaking it and the audience you have while completing it. Setting is important when we complete a task as different environments will have different associated pressures. Imagine having to intubate a patient in a hospital theatre before an emergency procedure—you are in a comfortable place, you have lots of equipment available and there are many people nearby who can help you if things go wrong. There are still pressures but they are more controlled, and you know there is less variability. Now imagine having to secure an airway on a patient at the side of the road after a car crash. It could be raining in winter, so you are wet and your hands are numb. You had to carry your bag of equipment down a steep embankment so you cannot easily get more from your response ambulance easily, and the equipment is limited. You are in a single crew response car and one of the first on the scene with very limited support if things go wrong. Both are emergencies but the latter setting has significantly increased pressures.

The way you are feeling can also play an important role in the pressures you experience when completing a task. We have all felt how much more difficult we find doing things when we are tired, unwell, upset or distracted by something else. Likewise, it is easier to feel more confident in what you are doing when you feel well rested, focused and engaged. Studies conducted by Ganesan et al. (2019) and Di Muzio et al. (2020) indicated that healthcare providers working shifts feel that they experience poorer quality sleep, feel more tired and exhibit decreased alertness and performance. The audience that is present can also lead to extra pressure when we carry out

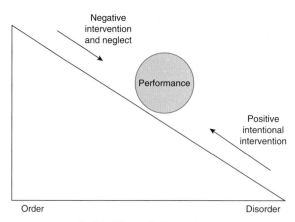

Fig. 2.3   Human factors entropy.

a task, causing us to second guess our judgment or doubt our skills. This sometimes leads people to try something new which is not in their usual practice, delay treatment to confirm something they already know or perform below their usual standards. Bodie (2010) acknowledged in a literature review the physiological and psychological effects of performing in front of an audience and how it can affect performance. In healthcare, it is common to have an audience, be that of our colleagues, a patient, their family or the general public; so it is important that we consider how to cope in these situations.

It is crucial from a human factors perspective that we make the effort to understand these pressures. By understanding the intrinsic and extrinsic pressures that affect the tasks we carry out, we can implement changes or mechanisms that help us cope with them and prevent errors. These mechanisms are, however, only effective with intentional effort. Ideally, we want to be in the flow level when we are working. We want to feel engaged in what we are doing and, when faced with a wave of challenges, have the knowledge and skills to surf along comfortably. Achieving this does not happen by accident and requires a number of positive human factors interventions and investments. A good way to think about it is to consider the physics concept of entropy. Entropy is a complicated concept but in basic terms it means that without intentional, concerted effort a system gradually declines into chaos. In a healthcare system, the decline could be caused by a culture of indifference to safety measures, gradual development of more and more shortcuts, staff not being able to attend courses to update their skills or low staffing leading to fatigue. To avoid the decline into 'chaos' we need to invest in ourselves, the people we lead and the organisations we manage (Fig. 2.3).

Strategies to Avoid Error

The aim of human factors in healthcare is to avoid errors occurring. There are many strategies that can help us avoid errors. Some will work in certain scenarios and others will not. For example, implementing a checklist could help structure a procedure and emphasise potential safety points. However, if the core issue is staff fatigue affecting work, a checklist may only have limited effect. Strategies are like tools in a toolbox; we need to use the correct one to fix the relevant problem. The strategies in the following sections are going to be split into three parts: personal, leadership and organisational. This is to help provide directed guidance depending on the positions we find ourselves in or problems we face (Fig. 2.4).

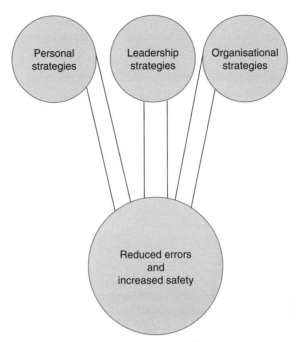

Fig. 2.4   Three sources of error avoidance strategy.

Personal

For an individual, there are a number of human factors strategies and practices we can adopt which can help us avoid errors.

Confidence and assertiveness can be very effective skills. Being confident in our own skills and knowledge can make us more effective, efficient and happier as a provider. This confidence should be in what you know but also in acknowledging what you do not know. Having the confidence to say you are at the boundary of your knowledge or abilities is not always an easy thing, especially when there are expectations of you. This confidence should be coupled with assertiveness, which is the ability to get your point across in a clear, direct manner. However, being assertive is not being aggressive or dominating, approaches that squash teamwork and collaboration (Arnold and Boggs, 2020). Tools such as CUS (concern-uncomfortable-safety) and DESC (describe-express-suggest-consequences (WHO, 2011) can be used to help promote and structure assertiveness skills. If we develop these skills, we can more easily acknowledge errors and improve safety.

A key way to gain confidence in your work is to improve your knowledge and experience through learning. In your working area, there will be opportunities for key learning which will help you to develop your skills and increase your confidence. This learning may be structured, such as courses and training regimes, or unstructured, such as area specific practices or experiences. Identifying and engaging in these opportunities will help you develop your skills as a healthcare provider.

Self-care has become an often-overused term and at times used as a substitute for larger scale change that would be difficult to implement. However, this does not detract from the fact that we as healthcare providers need to look after ourselves in order to work effectively. This can be anything from eating a balanced diet and exercising to making time for our mental health. Each person will have their own way to self-care or invest in their own wellbeing, but it is important that we do. Our jobs can be physically and mentally demanding, and so preparing ourselves is of great importance.

Amanda Astill: Emergency, General Ward and Maternity Unit Manager

Work–life balance is key. You need to have a job which you enjoy and leaves you with enough time and energy to come home, look after yourself and spend with the important people in your life. Finding the right balance is one of the most important things you can do in your life and will help make you safer at work.

Adopting an attitude of openness and learning at any level will help you to take advantage of the learning opportunities that arise and collaborate with those on your team. This can sometimes make us feel uncomfortable and vulnerable, especially for someone who has limited experience or confidence in their own skills. However, being able to open yourself up to new opinions or ways of doing things will drive your practice forward.

Leadership

Leadership in healthcare can take many forms. You may be an official leader with defined responsibilities or you may be an unofficial leader as a result of your knowledge and experience or circumstance. When we find ourselves in these positions, there are tools we can use to promote positive human factors and mitigate the possibilities for errors.

In most teams, there is a hierarchy which can be official or unofficial. Hierarchies, known in aerospace as a cockpit gradient, exist theoretically with a leader at the top who has the most knowledge and experience, and who cascades this down to the rest of the team and helps to effectively direct their activities. In real life, however, the leader may not always be the most knowledgeable and experienced team member in every situation. This does not necessarily detract from their position or skills in team management but does mean there needs to be a two-way flow of communication, be that of knowledge, views or experience. Flattening the hierarchy when there is a clear leader but also an environment where everyone can contribute equally can help avoid errors being made. Hearns (2019) suggests that some ways to foster this is to use team members' first names, make eye contact when communicating and adopt active listening techniques.

Hugh McDonald: Emergency Department Senior Charge Nurse

When you are leading a team, it is important to be approachable and open to discussion with your team. Making an effort to be fair, deescalate problems and engage your team in the department goals can be very effective. You should also try and balance the pressures experienced by your team with the expectations of those at higher levels. Part of your role is to balance the strategic goals with the real-world pressures and dynamics in your team.

Creating a shared mental model is another tool we can use to avoid human factors related errors. Our mental model is how were perceive a situation, what is important, what the focus is and what the dangers are. Depending on what we know or have experienced, this will be different for each team member. Diverging mental models can be common in emergency scenarios or where the care is complex and takes greater time. Without intervention, these divergent focuses can have a negative effect on the team's ability to achieve its collective goal. One way of helping to create a shared mental model is to actively pause, review what has happened, how everyone feels about it and what the plan is going ahead. An example of this is the surgical pause and checklist, a tool which has been implemented around the world and has improved patient safety greatly

(Clark et al., 2009; Haynes et al., 2009). Hearns (2019) adds that, when pausing, it is important to actively seek other team members' thoughts and opinions so as to create a supportive, flattened hierarchy. It is, however, important that this shared mental model helps direct the teams' focus rather than restricting it.

A key concept for any leader to be aware of is group think, coined by Janis (1972), which occurs when a team's mental model becomes so narrow that it is closed to possible alternative approaches and is hostile to disagreement. In this situation, team members can feel that the approval of the other team members is predicated on agreeing with the team's consensus and that this outweighs the importance of proposing a conflicting or alternative view. Some warning signs of this are when a team feels invulnerable to mistakes, collectively rationalises a course of action despite reasonable concerns being raised and holds stereotyped or harmful views of those who are not in the team (Arnold and Boggs, 2020). To avoid the group think trap, a leader could introduce new or temporary team members to give a fresh perspective. The leader could emphasise the importance of encouraging these and other team members' views openly, thus highlighting the value of honesty. They could also play the devil's advocate and disagree with the team, proposing an alternative opinion even if it is just to test the strength of the argument already discussed.

Organisational

Organisational implementation and support of positive human factors practices can have a significant effect on patient safety. The scope of change at an organisational level is much greater than that at a personal level. These changes can often be resource intensive and challenging to implement; however, when done effectively, can lead to safer and happier healthcare environments.

Considering how policy and practice guidelines affect human factors is an important step. Policies and guidelines may be negatively affecting human factors and need to be amended or they may have positive effects which could be replicated in other areas. Some examples include the adoption of safe patient–nurse ratios and mandating a rest period between shifts.

Another useful tool which can be used is analysing practices pre-emptively from a human factors perspective. This process of objectively looking at a practice and identifying the potential risk points and weaknesses can allow us to identify ways we can prevent them (McLeod and Bowie, 2018). A tool which has been used successfully for this purpose by the Royal Air Force is the bow-tie analysis (Ministry of Defence, 2014). This tool maps hazardous practices and the events that can occur; then, it identifies the threats, contributing factors and consequences and the barriers in place to prevent errors from occurring (Fig. 2.5).

A final organisational step is to create a supportive culture and environment for staff and patients. This is a challenging and multifaceted goal to achieve and there is no silver bullet. Fostering a culture which is open to critique, supportive of learning and willing to make changes is an important step to reducing errors. For example, reducing the number of clinical hours nurses work to allow them to complete training, such as team-based simulation training. This would require investment in the training itself as well as resources to cover staff to allow them to attend training without disrupting the provision of care.

What to Do When an Error Occurs

Errors in healthcare are a complex and highly emotional subject. We, and the people we care for, expect a high level of knowledge, competence and professionalism. The healthcare industry, like many other safety critical industries, is focused on consistently providing the best outcomes. When an error does occur, it can be a challenging event for everyone. Putting aside malicious and

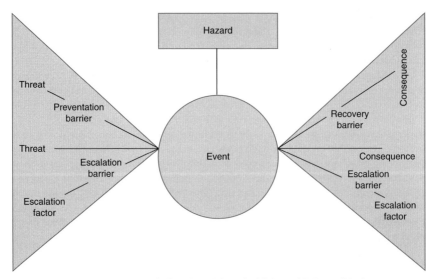

Fig. 2.5　Bowtie analysis; adapted from the Ministry of Defence (2014).

negligent acts, healthcare providers who have worked hard to gather the skills and knowledge vital to safe practice are invested in the care they provide. It is important that we support these providers and foster a system that effectively learns from mistakes and replicates positive experiences.

When an error happens our first priority is patient welfare: rectifying the error, monitoring the patient for ill effects and involving the required professionals in a time sensitive fashion. Afterwards, the incident needs to be reported. Different organisations have their own mechanisms and policies for reporting errors or near misses. It is the duty of the provider to report the error, even if they share the blame in part or in entirety. This duty of honesty and candour is of great importance for any healthcare professional. However, there is also a responsibility for those being reported too, to carefully consider the error and its causes. A reported error should be analysed in a way that carefully studies the incident, what contributed to it occurring and fairly identify actions which can be taken to avoid its reoccurrence. One element of achieving this is to adopt a just culture, wherein responsibility is fairly judged and apportioned (Boysen, 2013). In a just culture, a professional is responsible for practicing in a safe way, but when an incident occurs the focus is not on apportioning blame but analysing what went wrong; for example, when a medication error occurs, the focus is to analyse the events that led up to it and how to address them. This may include identifying a personal error by the person who dispensed the drug but would equally consider the other factors, such as whether the prescribing system was flawed, the medication packaging was confusing or if the same mistake had been made before. By doing this, we can not only highlight opportunities for personal development but also effectively identify areas to make the system safer for everyone.

Flt Lt Matt Douglas: RAF Fast Jet Pilot

When conducting complex tasks during high pressure and dynamic situations, it is inevitable that errors or incorrect decisions will be made at some point. When this happens, it is important to acknowledge it, rectify the error where possible and then focus back on the mission with full attention. Dwelling on the error will only lead to more serious mistakes being made and potentially risk mission success.

Reflection and debriefing are a key part of the analysis process when an error occurs. Norris and Lockey (2012) identified reflection and debriefing as key tools for improving team knowledge, skills and working in resuscitation. Having those involved take the time to talk through what happened, why it happened and how they feel about it is a useful and effective tool. It is not uncommon when healthcare providers open up about errors that they made to talk about the profound negative emotions connected to the incident. Words like 'shame', 'embarrassment', 'remorse' and 'worst fears realised' are common during these conversations, even when the conversations are few and far between. It is hard to admit to an error and harder still to confront the emotions. These negative emotions can indicate that the person is experiencing the second victim phenomenon. This occurs when a person made a mistake which actually did or potentially could have caused harm to someone in their care and feels significant negative emotions which damage their mental health (Dekker, 2013). Dekker (2013) highlights that while the vast majority of research considers that the negative effects of second victimhood come from healthcare, there is very little written about how to effectively address it, suggesting that this is a problem in healthcare that we are not appropriately addressing. Dekker and Breakey (2016) acknowledge the importance of reflection and debriefing in addressing the needs of 'second victims' and in helping to build self-resilience, something which is essential to organisation resilience.

Conclusion

This chapter has considered the concept of human error as well as its potential impact and associated learning. It has also highlighted options for what to do when an error occurs. In healthcare, it is essential to be Conscious that errors occur because we are humans and we make mistakes. Our overarching aim is to reduce error by mitigating risk. In this chapter, we have offered examples of incidents and contextualised strategies to minimise recurrence of similar events.

Key Points
- Errors do happen but we can actively work to prevent them.
- To avoid errors we need to consider human factors at an individual, leadership and organisational level.
- Without positive, intentional intervention, performance and safety will decline.
- When an error does occur we have a responsibility to examine and learn from it without focus on blame.

References

Arnold, E., Boggs, K.U., 2020. Interpersonal Relationships: Professional Communication Skills for Nurses, eighth ed. Saunders, Philadelphia.

Bodie, G.D., 2010. A racing heart, rattling knees, and ruminative thoughts: defining, explaining, and treating public speaking anxiety. Commun. Educ. 59 (1), 70–105.

Boysen, P.G., 2013. Just culture: a foundation for balanced accountability and patient safety. Ochsner J. 13 (3), 400–406.

Carayon, P., Wetterneck, T.B., Rivera-Rodriguez, A.J., Hundt, A.S., Hoonakker, P., Holden, R., et al., 2014. Human factors systems approach to healthcare quality and patient safety. Appl. Ergon. 45 (1), 14–25.

Clark, E., Squire, S., Heyme, A., Mickle, M.E., Petrie, E., 2009. The PACT Project: improving communication at handover. Med. J. Aust. 190 (11), S125–S127.

Dekker, S., 2013. Second Victim: Error, Guilt, Trauma, and Resilience, first ed. CRC Press, Boca Raton.

Dekker, S.W., Breakey, H., 2016. 'Just culture': improving safety by achieving substantive, procedural and restorative justice. Saf. Sci. 85, 187–193.

Di Muzio, M., Diella, G., Di Simone, E., Novelli, L., Alfonsi, V., Scarpelli, S., et al., 2020. Nurses and night shifts: poor sleep quality exacerbates psychomotor performance. Front. Neurosci. 14, 579938.

Diamond, D.M., 2005. Cognitive, endocrine and mechanistic perspectives on non-linear relationships between arousal and brain function. Nonlinearity Biol. Toxicol. Med. 3 (1), 1–7.

Ganesan, S., Magee, M., Stone, J.E., Mulhall, M.D., Collins, A., Howard, M.E., et al., 2019. The impact of shift work on sleep, alertness and performance in healthcare workers. Sci. Rep. 9 (1), 4635.

Haddon-Cave, C., 2009. The Nimrod Review. The Stationary Office, London.

Hall, L.H., Johnson, J., Watt, I., Tsipa, A., O'Connor, D.B., 2016. Healthcare staff wellbeing, burnout, and patient safety: a systematic review. PLoS One 11 (7), e0159015.

Haynes, A.B., Weiser, T.G., Berry, W.R., Lipsitz, S.R., Breizat, A.H., Dellinger, E.P., et al., 2009. A surgical safety checklist to reduce morbidity and mortality in a global population. N. Engl. J. Med. 360 (5), 491–499.

Hearns, S., 2019. Peak Performance Under Pressure: Lessons from a Helicopter Rescue Doctor. Class Professional Publishing, Bridgwater.

Institute of Medicine (US), 2000. Committee on quality of health care in America. In: Kohn, L.T., Corrigan, J.M., Donaldson, M.S. (Eds.), To Err Is Human: Building a Safer Health System. National Academies Press (US), Washington, D.C.

International Atomic Energy Agency, 1992. The Chernobyl Accident: Updating of INSAG-I (INSAG-7). International Atomic Energy Agency, Vienna.

Janis, I.L., 1972. Victims of Groupthink: A Psychological Study of Foreign-Policy Decisions and Fiascos. Houghton, Mifflin, Boston.

Kelly, F.E., Frerk, C., Bailey, C.R., Cook, T.M., Ferguson, K., Flin, R., et al., 2023. Implementing human factors in anaesthesia: guidance for clinicians, departments and hospitals. Anaesthesia 78 (4), 458–478.

McLeod, R.W., Bowie, P., 2018. Bowtie Analysis as a prospective risk assessment technique in primary healthcare. Policy Pract. Health Saf. 16 (2), 177–193.

Mendl, M., 1999. Performing under pressure: stress and cognitive function. Appl. Anim. Behav. Sci. 65 (3), 221–244.

Mid Staffordshire NHS Foundation Trust Public Inquiry, 2013. Report of the Mid Staffordshire-NHS Foundation Trust Public Inquiry. The Stationery Office, London.

Ministry of Defence, 2014. Manual of Air Safety (MAS). Ministry of Defence, London.

National Quality Board, 2013. Human Factors in Healthcare: A Concordat from the National Quality Board. National Quality Board, London.

Norris, E.M., Lockey, A.S., 2012. Human factors in resuscitation teaching. Resuscitation 83 (4), 423–427.

Parker, S.H., 2015. Human factors science: brief history and applications to healthcare. Curr. Probl. Pediatr. Adolesc. Health Care 45 (12), 390–394.

Plokhy, S., 2018. Chernobyl: History of a Tragedy. Penguin Books UK, London.

Presidential Commission on the Space Shuttle Challenger Accident, 1986. Report of the Presidential Commission on the Space Shuttle Challenger Accident. Government Printing Office, Washington, D.C.

Roth, C., Brewer, M., Wieck, K.L., 2017. Using a Delphi method to identify human factors contributing to nursing errors. Nurs. Forum 52 (3), 173–179.

Russ, A.L., Weiner, M., Saleem, J.J., Wears, R.L., 2012. When 'technically preventable' alerts occur, the design—not the prescriber—has failed. J. Am. Med. Inform. Assoc. 19 (6), 1119–1120.

Russ, A.L., Fairbanks, R.J., Karsh, B.T., Militello, L.G., Saleem, J.J., Wears, R.L., 2013. The science of human factors: separating fact from fiction. BMJ Qual. Saf. 22 (10), 802–808.

Sandi, C., 2013. Stress and cognition. Wiley Interdiscip Rev Cogn Sci. 4 (3), 245–261.

Scanlon, M.C., Karsh, B.T., 2010. Value of human factors to medication and patient safety in the intensive care unit. Crit. Care Med. 38 (6 Suppl. l), S90S96.

Tingle, J., 2011. The WHO patient safety curriculum guide. Br. J. Nurs. 20 (22), 1456–1457.

Wilson, J.R., 2014. Fundamentals of systems ergonomics/human factors. Appl. Ergon. 45 (1), 5–13.

World Health Organization, 2011. Patient Safety Curriculum Guide. World Health Organization, Geneva.

Yerkes, R.M., Dodson, J.D., 1908. The relation of strength of stimulus to rapidity of habit-formation. J. Comp. Neurol. Psychol. 18 (5), 459–482.

Patient Safety

Karon Cormack

Introduction

Achieving patient safety is the desire of every healthcare professional because keeping patients safe from harm is fundamental for the provision of good quality care. Our purpose is to improve the condition of those we treat, to the best of our clinical abilities and modern medicine, and not cause more illness or injury.

Our attitude towards harm preventability has thankfully changed over the years. In the past, harm from hospital acquired infection (HAI), pressure ulcers and falls were deemed unavoidable; however, we have learned that much can be done to facilitate reduction of the occurrence of such predictable events.

The attitude of the public towards healthcare has also changed because people are generally better informed, have greater expectations and are less tolerant. Patients and relatives feel more empowered to ask questions and are less accepting when things go wrong. The level of complaints has been significantly greater than in the past 5 years, and patients and relatives more often request copies of their medical records to see what has been written about their care. This should not be considered negatively, because each complaint should be viewed as a gift to provide insight for improvement. Patient opinions on what is expected and acceptable are good drivers for quality and raise the standards of care.

Management of Patient Safety

AVOIDING

Implementing established and proven systems and methods to reduce the chances of known harms occurring is fundamental to patient safety. These could be clinical standards and guidelines or protocols and standard operating procedures that keep staff on the right track to avoid known harms.

These interventions can range from something very generic, such as hand washing, which will have a significant influence on HAI, to something specific, like a swab and instrument policy, to prevent retained objects during surgical operations.

For avoidance of these known harms to be successful requires not just issue awareness but also accurate implementation of a proposed solution. For solutions to be implemented correctly, we must consider human factors and make it easy to do so. For example, imagine a 12 bed area with patients who need a significant amount of 'hands on' interventions requiring regular handwashing by the staff. There is only one sink in the ward at bed one—how easy will it be to keep washing your hands when working at bed 12, while working alongside your colleagues who are required to use the same sink? Hospital designs have changed, in recognition of HAI influence, to accommodate more single rooms, each with their own sink and en suite facilities. This is ergonomics (also called human factors) in action to reduce cross infection between patients. Modifications in designs to improve performance can be an excellent way to alter behaviour because changes in environment or equipment can almost force a person to do the right thing.

Similarly, for a swab and instrument policy to be followed correctly, the infrastructure requires the presence of items such as a visible board to record the count, staff available to perform a two-person count and equipment to display the swabs.

This becomes apparent when investigating events that should have been avoided but still happened. These events are generally called Never Events due to the perception that because we know exactly what to do to avoid these events, they should never happen (Table 3.1).

Therefore, the retention of a surgical swab is a Never Event because if the protocols and policies relating to counting swabs are followed, the event is avoided. However sometimes the assumption of the Never Event is not as clear cut as in an operating theatre procedure, which has been designed with this practice in mind with swab boards, racks and books to accommodate the counting. There is a designated scrub nurse and a circulating nurse who have the responsibility of counting and tracking all the swabs. In contrast, a labour suite delivery room may not contain the same infrastructure. There is an assumption that if open operative treatments are required, the patient would be transferred to the operating theatre; other smaller procedures are low risk for swab retention. However, the critical nature of obstetric cases can escalate very quickly to the point that a lone mid wife is assisting an obstetrician who requires surgical instruments and swabs rapidly for a deteriorating patient with heavy bleeding. There has been no count of the swabs at the beginning, there is no board to mark them on and there is no one else to help count; blood

---

TABLE 3.1 ■ **Never Events List**

Wrong surgery site: invasive procedure on the wrong patient or at the wrong site
Wrong implant/prosthesis: implant/prosthesis different from that planned
Retained foreign object post procedure: swab, instruments, catheters, etc.
Misselection of a strong potassium solution: intravenous strong potassium solution
Medication given by the wrong route: e.g. intravenous chemotherapy by the intrathecal route
Overdose of insulin due to abbreviations or incorrect device: 10-fold or greater
Overdose of methotrexate for noncancer treatment: using electronic prescribing
Misselection of high strength midazolam during conscious sedation: e.g. 5mg/ml
Failure to install functional collapsible shower/curtain rails: mental health inpatient
Falls from poorly restricted windows: within reach of patients
Chest or neck entrapment in bed rails: with equipment provided by the National Health Service.
Transfusion or transplantation of ABO-incompatible blood components or organs
Misplaced naso- or orogastric tubes: not detected before feed, flush or medication
Scalding of patients: scalded by water used for washing/bathing
Unintentional connection of a patient requiring oxygen to an air flowmeter

National Health Service Improvement, 2018

sodden swabs are on the instrument tray, on the floor, in the bin and quite possibly inside the patient. Even the most traumatic theatre cases do not have this level of chaos, as the systems for safety are embedded in the procedures. A retained swab, regardless of where it occurs, is still a Never Event because we know what we need to put in place to avoid this; however, in some situations, we do not always do it.

The study of human factors aims to improve human performance of tasks considering all the elements that would influence success. Although a policy is a good step towards providing instructions, it is useless if the staff are not trained in how to perform, the infrastructure is not present to support compliance and there is a culture of ignoring the rules. Therefore, Never Events still occur. Circumstances conspire against the staff members, creating conditions that make compliance with the recommended system impossible.

However, having a list of Never Events is still a good idea because by identifying these events we can monitor them and recognise when there has been failure. This creates the opportunity to change the system by strengthening the interventions required to support better compliance and reduce occurrence.

National Health Service Improvement has chosen 15 events to qualify as Never Events; however, it is important to note the description details, because not all aspects of each topic are considered avoidable, as the systems to prevent it are not in place (Table 3.1). For example, scalding is on the list, but only when it is related to bathing (e.g. placing a patient in a scalding hot bath); it does not include spilt hot drinks or other potential scenarios.

RISK

Healthcare providers have a duty under the Health and Safety at Work Regulations (1999) to identify what might cause harm to patients and staff. These are known as hazards and can relate to different factors such as the environment, equipment, procedures and substances. Risk is defined as the combination of how likely and how serious the harm would be if the hazard occurred. If the hazard cannot be removed, then the requirement is to control or mitigate it. To help quantify risk, a risk matrix can be used which looks at the assessments of likelihood and severity and indicates a score defining the risk as low, medium or high. Previous clinical trials provided clinicians with estimated risks relating to clinical procedures, usually described as a percentage or a rate, which can aid decision making.

Risk assessment is also a way of reducing the occurrence or impact of a known threat. This process identifies a hazard, considers who could be harmed and evaluates the risk and what can be done to prevent the impact. The risk is evaluated by considering how likely it is to occur and what the impact would be if it did occur.

Traditionally, risk assessment is thought of as a method to prevent hazards in a workplace and would be part of a health and safety toolkit. However, in healthcare, there are numerous clinical risk assessments that are designed to assess the risk to a patient in relation to a range of particular topics such as falls, nutrition or suicide. For example, the Bowtie diagram is a versatile tool for displaying and understanding risks and effects, and can help effectively manage unsafe acts and critical incidents (Culwick et al., 2020).

This type of risk assessment usually consists of a series of questions that lead to a score which, in turn, would indicate a suggested care plan. This not only helps to identify potential problems before they occur so they can be prevented, but also helps to standardise care and treatment.

Although these risk assessments are helpful, if they increase significantly in number, frequency and complexity, they can become burdensome and would be completed in a mechanistic way with little thought. If this occurs, the effectiveness of the tool is depleted—resulting in errors in the assessment. Therefore, it is wise to tailor each clinical risk assessment for patients that would benefit from them so that the appropriate time is taken to produce the correct care pathway.

Human factors influence this situation, because if the staff thinks that the task they are doing is worthwhile, there is more chance they will perform it to a high standard. It is a compromise between performing the same risk assessment on all patients with the chance of identifying an issue in very few patients (that would otherwise not have been identified) or selecting a smaller cohort of patients that will gain more benefit from the risk assessment—for example, performing a falls risk assessment on every single patient or limiting it to those who meet initial criteria such as age, previous fall history and particular clinical conditions prone to falling. Another factor to be considered is the time it takes to perform the risk assessments and whether it is realistic to expect nursing staff to complete a significant amount of paperwork thoroughly in a restricted time-frame. In summary, if it is well-designed and straightforward to complete, limited to the cohort of patients who would benefit from them and staff are given the time to complete it correctly, risk assessments are a very useful tool in identifying patient safety requirements.

This is one example of a risk assessment tool; many are available free via the Internet. There are many examples of risk assessment tools.

> *'Work-As-Imagined describes what should happen under normal working conditions. Work-As-Done, on the other hand, describes what actually happens, how work unfolds over time in complex contexts'.*
>
> **Hollnagel et al., 2015**

Another element to consider here is the work of Hollnagel et al. (2015) regarding the difference between 'work imagined' and 'work done' which emphasises the difference between looking at a work procedure on paper and watching it being performed (Fig. 3.1). A simple example would be the number of nursing procedures that include checking a patient name band; however, when observing procedures, particular action is not always followed. There can be many reasons the action was not done, such as deeming the check unnecessary as the nurses feel that they know the patient, lack of time or the name band was not put on in the first place. If the gap between the written procedure and the practice is too wide, a comprehensive understanding of human factors and behaviour is required. Just reminding staff that they should be doing something will not achieve success because the reasons for the noncompliance must be explored—the procedure could be unrealistic, the staff might feel elements are not required and waste time or the required kit is unavailable or insufficient. Examining these human factors will unlock the key to what needs to be done for improvement. The differences in policy and practice also highlight the need for engagement with the people doing the task and consideration of their operational and clinical environments. A manager or committee who are distant from the 'shop floor' will not have the insights required to ensure what is being asked in a policy is realistic and achievable.

There also needs to be a degree of flexibility in policies and procedures due to the many variables clinical staff are dealing with simultaneously. Healthcare is different from other industries that can be totally mechanised or completely protocol-driven due to the number of variables that can happen in a day or even in a task. Healthcare staff develop an amazing set of skills to navigate all the system inadequacies, unexpected challenges and variability to still achieve good patient

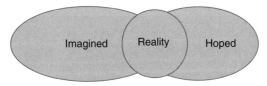

Fig. 3.1   Diagram representing work as imagined versus work as done and the reality.

care. Hollnagel et al. (2015) would advocate celebrating this and learning not only when tasks go wrong but also when they go right.

Involving patients in their own healthcare can also be a useful way to enable patient safety.

> 'Patients are uniquely qualified to share views and identify issues with their care, given they are present throughout that care'.
> **National Health Service Improvement, 2021**

Encouraging patients to ask questions and to raise concerns can prevent an adverse event. Can you imagine the relief if you are administering medication and a wrong drug incident is avoided because the patient said 'my pill at this time of the day is usually blue, not pink'?

However, we need to create the conditions that make patients and their relatives comfortable to speak up, ask why something has changed in the treatment plan or if there are alternatives to the treatment planned. It is helpful to openly share information with patients so that they can be involved in monitoring their symptoms and be more informed about their medications.

Some hospitals have been proactive in this regard and provide patients with leaflets, question prompt cards or an animated video to watch so the patient knows what patient safety issues to watch out for. Patients have been an untapped resource in the past and perceived as passive passengers on their own treatment journey; however, involving them benefits not only the patient but also the staff as patient safety is improved.

IMPROVEMENT

Patient safety programmes to improve systems of care have been established in the United Kingdom for over 10 years. The origins of this work came from the Institute of Healthcare Improvement (IHI) in the United States of America, founded by Don Berwick who built on methodologies in industry to apply to healthcare (see https://www.ihi.org/ for relevant papers). The main contribution to the IHI approach is the work of Edward Deming, who devised the Lens of Profound Knowledge (Langley et al., 2009) (Fig. 3.2). This is a methodology that encourages more understanding and analysis of the system to be improved before embarking on implementing what may be perceived as a good idea. This model contains four areas defined as lenses with which to view service improvement activity: 1) appreciating a system, 2) understanding variation, 3) psychology and 4) the theory of knowledge.

The concept is that before you can improve a system you need to really understand how it currently works and what influences success by looking at who performs the task, why they do it the way they currently do and whether everyone is doing it the same way. The aim is to develop theories that will improve processes and subsequent outcomes by standardising processes.

This model of improvement is widely used as the chosen method to consider the elements required for successful improvement by testing the theories. The focus is on small scale testing using the plan-do-study-act model, so that changes to the process can be tested in real work settings and frequently adjusted to achieve the greatest success.

Patient safety improvement work identifies heath care topics known to cause potential harm that respond to interventions known to lead to improvement. It is important to not confuse this with innovation as the interventions had already been researched and shown to be effective. Some of these interventions are called an improvement bundle because they are a collection of individual elements that have the greatest impact if performed together for each patient. Some of these bundles have become standard practice—such as the ventilator associated pneumonia bundle which includes intensive care patients having a 30-degree tilt bed position—and the implementation of some are still underway—such as the stroke bundle (collection of elements that improve

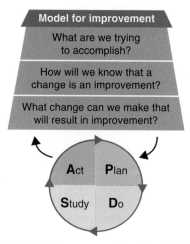

Fig. 3.2 Model for improvement (Langley et al., 2009).

outcomes of patients with stroke) and sepsis six (immediate care to be given with suspected sepsis to improve outcome).

Part of the improvement methodology is to measure the process and if possible, the outcomes. These measurements are performed over time and displayed in run charts or process control charts to identify if the process measures are being successfully implemented. For example, if the change idea was to improve communication by implementing a team huddle, the occurrence of the huddle could be recorded each day. This would allow further analysis of the days on which it did not occur and finding out what happened to prevent the huddle that day. A test of change could be to modify the time of the huddle and assess if that improved occurrence. These data can be used to show staff their performance and can provide an incentive to improve. However, this is only of value if the staff believe the change is worthwhile, otherwise sharing and displaying data will not have the desired effect.

As previously mentioned, the psychology of those performing the task is one of the lenses required for improvement. This is crucial because changing behaviour can be very difficult especially when staff are busy with many other demands. Some of the reasons change is difficult include staff habitually doing tasks the same way, more effort is required to change and if the staff does not feel the need to change. The human factors element of the improvement model is crucial because for any change to be sustainable the hearts and minds of the staff performing the task need to be engaged; they not only need to understand what to do but also believe it is the right thing to do. Otherwise, they will cut corners, deviate from the process or revert to the 'old way' of performing the task.

As time passes and an improvement becomes more embedded it becomes culturally more and more unacceptable to do things the 'old way'. For example, in the past, nursing staff would frequently manually lift patients. The method of manual lifting changed over time, but it was still manual lifting and this not only caused injury to the patients but also damaged the health of the nurses. Hoists were brought in as the solution to the problem, but in the beginning they were bulky and unwieldy, often only one per ward; therefore, it took longer to lift a patient and it required more effort. Although a solution was provided and it protected the nurses, it still took time to stop the nurses from manually lifting because it was quicker and they did not have time to use the solution. In addition, when you are young and fit, you are perhaps not thinking about what damage you are doing to your back and what you will be like after 20 years of lifting. However, it is now culturally unacceptable to manually lift in the manner which was commonplace in the past. The culture of what is acceptable and what is common practice has changed.

One of the success factors in implementing patient safety initiatives is to work with and listen to the staff who perform the task related to the improvement. This is when testing the change ideas is vital. The need to alter and adapt the original plan to encourage adoption is key. This also relates to making it easier to do the right thing. Even when designing forms, charts and care plans, it is vital to test before the final version is adopted. Too often, a committee can take months over several meetings designing the perfect form, only to find that when it hits the 'shop floor' the staff really dislike it—for example, the way to complete it does not flow, a box is too small for the information required, a question is ambiguous or there is repetition. The people designing the form are often not the people who will be completing it. Involving the staff and listening to their ideas for change and improvement will enhance engagement and commitment, and encourage them to show the extra effort required to make the change.

> 'We all make errors irrespective of how much training and experience we possess or how motivated we are to do it right. Failures are more serious for jobs where the consequences of errors are not protected'.
>
> **Management of Health and Safety at Work Regulations, 1999**

Learning from Adverse Events

Knowledge regarding the sources of error has improved over the past 30 years. There is a better understanding that adverse events are not the sole responsibility of a frontline worker without organisational control. The recognition of human factors and responsibility of the organisation to consider them are required to control risks and improve safety (Management of Health and Safety at Work Regulations, 1999).

There has been a change in thinking, from viewing the workers as the root of the problem due to their inattention, carelessness and negligence to recognising that the source of errors are more often related to conditions and circumstances that the workers endure.

When an adverse event occurs, the first priority is to attend to the patient to reduce the impact, and if possible, provide remedy or further treatment as required. This could be anything from providing a naloxone hydrochloride for an opioid overdose, resuscitation following deterioration or an X-ray following a fall to assess for fractures. However, not all adverse events are realised at the time they occur as an error may be realised sometime later. For example, when reviewing the patient records after a patient deteriorated, it was discovered that observations were missed or the early warning score was wrongly calculated; thus, earlier intervention could have prevented the decline in health.

Regardless of when the incident occurred and was discovered, it is important to have an open and honest conversation with the patient and in some circumstances, their relatives. It is important to acknowledge what happened and apologise for it. There can be a reluctance to apologise if there is a lack of understanding at the time of how and why the event happened. If this is the case, it is better to explain you are sorry for what happened and that you will be looking into it to understand why it occurred.

If we are to develop a trusting relationship with patients, we must have an open dialogue when things go wrong. Patients have a right to know what happened and how this will influence their health. Although there has always been a professional duty of candour to be honest with patients regarding their treatment options, complications and prognosis, there is a legal requirement for duty of candour when a serious adverse event occurs. It is quite common for patients and relatives who have experienced an adverse event to say that their motivation for answers is that they do not want this to happen to someone else. Similarly, as healthcare providers, we should remember that adverse events and complaints provide an opportunity for valuable learning.

To gain learning from adverse events, we need to understand how and why the event happened by investigating. The quality of the investigation will dictate the level of learning possible. It is much easier to explain what happened and how it happened by describing the steps that lead up to the event, but if we are to learn we also need to understand why it happened. To do this, we must consider assessing the human factors in relation to the event.

There are two main groups of errors. Active errors occur at the level of the frontline operator with the effects being felt almost immediately. These would result in an act (something that was done that should not have been done) or an omission (something not done that should have been done). Latent errors tend to be removed from the direct control of the operator and include historical, background issues such as poor design and poor management decisions. When analysing adverse events, both types of errors require consideration.

There can be numerous elements that influence a human to perform a task, especially in a complex environment such as healthcare where staff have multiple goals and competing demands. It is vital to look at the systemic issues rather than concentrate on the individual. It is very rare that a rogue staff member is the only cause of an adverse event; even in such cases, it is often observed that any staff member working in similar circumstances could perform the same error. Therefore, it is of no benefit to punish and 'make an example' of those who perform errors as the conditions that created the error are still there waiting for the next opportunity to cause a problem. For the same reason, it is foolhardy to believe that we will prevent errors by encouraging staff to try harder or constantly reminding them of what should be done, without changing the system.

There are several helpful tools that can help to determine potential human factors. The Systems Engineering Initiative for Patient Safety (SEIPS) model (NHS England, 2021) identifies key components of work systems, work processes and work outcomes (Fig. 1.2).

The work systems include elements that are connected and relate to each other, and are therefore interdependent. These elements are people, environments, tools and tasks. The work processes are about how the work is performed and who performs it. Work outcomes are the results from the combination of the previous two which could be wanted or unwanted. The arrows in the model represent the causal feedback loops. This model is not only useful for analysing a system as part of an adverse event investigation but also has uses when designing services or quality improvement work.

Most significant adverse events occur from a catalogue of system issues that accumulate to create the conditions for error. Common circumstances could be:

- Shortness of time (short staffing, inadequate skill mix)
- Staff unfamiliar with the environment (bank, agency, redeployed staff)
- Staff required to work beyond their level of competence
- New or complex equipment
- Lack of supervision
- Lack of experience
- Unexpected change to the routine or process
- Undefined team roles
- Unfamiliar team (no time to develop trust or competency awareness)
- Unfamiliar tasks to be performed

These examples are not a definitive list; there are many more risk-prone circumstances that we can find ourselves in that will increase the likelihood of error. Being aware that these circumstances can put our practice at risk can help to avoid an incident from occurring.

A good analogy: you would not drive the same way in a heavy snowfall with poor visibility and slippery roads as you would on a clear day. You would recognise the environment you are in is difficult, and therefore you would moderate your speed and increase your level of concentration and alertness. When system issues accumulate in healthcare, staff appear less likely to moderate their work patterns and try and work faster to accommodate everything they are required to do when the system is more stable (normal condition). When feeling overwhelmed, it is difficult to take a minute to stand back and prioritise tasks, delegate or ask for help because our default is to be self-reliant and cope. Unfortunately, the more we cope, the more tolerance we build for these risk-prone conditions, and it is only a matter of time until an error occurs which can result in an adverse event—just as if you do not reduce your speed or increase your concentration when driving in bad weather, you will be more likely to skid and cause an accident.

Several key elements need to be in place to effectively investigate an adverse event. A robust investigation is usually reserved for events that resulted in a very poor patient outcome such as death, serious injury or ill health; reviews can be time consuming and require a certain level of training and understanding. However, it must be recognised that patient outcome can be a matter of chance, and therefore we should also investigate events that could have caused a serious outcome. For example, if a patient was given what could be considered a fatal dose of a medication, such as insulin or an opioid and the patient actually survived, learning from investigating may prevent an actual fatality. This scenario can be referred to as a near miss.

The term 'near miss' can cover two different scenarios. One is where an error or omission occurred which could have caused harm to a patient, member of staff or others, but fortunately in this instance there was no adverse outcome (such as in the example in the previous paragraph). The term 'near miss' does not actually describe what happened because, if you think about it, it was actually a 'hit' because the event happened but did not cause harm.

The other description for near miss applies when the error was about to take place and a last minute intervention, either by chance or design, prevented the incident from occurring. For example, there was a medication prescription error, but it was identified just before administration. The term 'near miss' is more accurate here as the event did not happen.

Reports of near miss events are helpful because they identify the same weaknesses in the system that would cause an adverse outcome, without the harm being caused; therefore, they are a rich source of learning about adverse events resulting in harm.

Investigating significant adverse events requires individuals performing the review to be trained. They need to understand the process and have a good understanding of organisational policy and procedures. They also need to have a knowledge of human factors and skills in interviewing and report writing.

To investigate an adverse event, numerous sources of evidence will be gathered that relate to the event including investigating the staff and departments that were part of the patient care. The staff involved are eyewitnesses and the strongest source of evidence. Staff may be required to a write a recollection of events that would provide an account of their actions. For key staff closely involved in the event, it may be helpful to interview them because this provides richer information and the opportunity to ask questions.

It is understandable that staff may have feelings of worry and guilt when involved in an event that has resulted in patient harm and concerns about their employment and reputation. It is very important that staff feel that they are supported throughout the investigation process. This support can take many forms including:

- Debriefing following the event (as a staff group or individually)
- Keeping staff informed of the investigation process (timescales)
- Explaining what will be expected of staff with respect to the investigation
- Treating staff kindly when interviewing by being attentive, understanding and using a cognitive interview technique
- Explaining whether a report will be written and what will happen to the report

It is good practice for investigators to anonymise reports and provide staff involved with the opportunity to comment on the draft before the final version. Staff worry what will be written about them and how they will be portrayed in the report; hence, if assurance can be given that they will have the opportunity to read it, some anxieties can be eliminated.

Other sources of information related to the event may be policies, guidelines, standard operating procedures, a device manual, medication indication or posology. This collection of evidence relates to what is expected to occur to be able to identify any difference from what actually occurred.

The investigation should then identify, analyse and prioritise the key issues that have a causal relationship to the outcome using tools such as the SEIPS model previously described.

Each report should have a conclusion that provides a clear summary of why the event occurred and if it could have been prevented, which should link to any recommendations that follow. Recommendations require to be actionable rather than a vague desire for something to improve or a statement of fact about the clinical process.

The easiest recommendations to implement are often the weakest in terms of impact on the problem. For example, an investigation revealed that there was a problem with handover between two clinical areas because a vital piece of information regarding patient allergy was not communicated to the receiving area. An easy recommendation would be to 'remind all staff to include patient allergies when handing over'. A better recommendation would be to look at the handover form and ask staff what could be done with it to make it easier to record this important information. Is there a specific question prompt about this? If there is, is it in an obvious place? Would it help to have key questions in a different coloured box? Redesigning the form to make it easier to record allergies will have more influence on staff behaviour than sending out reminders. Staff want to get it right, but because humans can be distracted, interrupted and tired we need the systems we work in to be as easy as possible to help maintain good practice when the going gets tough.

> '...the definition of safety should be changed from "avoiding that something goes wrong" to "ensuring that everything goes right." Safety-II is the system's ability to function as required under varying conditions, so that the number of intended and acceptable outcomes (in other words, everyday activities) is as high as possible'.
>
> **Hollnagel et al., 2015**

Conclusion

Although we can learn from when 'things go wrong', we can also learn from when 'things go right'. There is as much to learn from examining why, a majority of the time, an issue did not occur even though the same latent factors were present. This is referred to as a Safety-II approach that describes the ability to still succeed in task or performance despite the varying conditions in the working environment. This line of thinking appreciates the flexibility and resilience of staff to adapt and still achieve their goal while responding to system shortfalls and surprises. Therefore, a combination of learning from adverse events (Safety-I) combined with an appreciation and review of how success is normally achieved (Safety-II) (MacKinnon et al., 2021) will provide more insights to employ improvements.

To achieve patient safety, healthcare staff are required to be intentional in their behaviour in relation to avoiding or improving potential patient safety issues and learning when a patient safety issue has occurred. Patient safety does not happen by accident.

Key Points

Considerations for you, your team and your organisation:
- Look at the system as a whole.
- How do you learn from previous incidences?
- How do you share learnings?
- What is your attitude towards safety?
- Do you have a culture of safety?

References

Culwick, M.D., Endlich, Y., Prineas, S.N., 2020. The Bowtie diagram: a simple tool for analysis and planning in anesthesia. Curr. Opin. Anaesthesiol. 33 (6), 808–814.

Health and Safety at Work Regulations, 1999. https://www.legislation.gov.uk/uksi/1999/3242/contents/made [hard return].

Holden, R.J., Carayon, P., 2021. SEIPS 101 and seven simple SEIPS tools. BMJ Qual. Saf. 30 (11), 901–910.

Hollnagel, E., Wears, R.L., Braithwaite, J., 2015. From safety-I to safety-II: a white paper. In: The Resilient Health Care Net: Published Simultaneously by the University of Southern Denmark. University of Florida, USA, and Macquarie University, Australia.

Langley, G.L., Moen, R., Nolan, K.M., Nolan, T.W., Norman, C.L., Provost, L.P., 2009. The Improvement Guide: A Practical Approach to Enhancing Organizational Performance, second ed. Jossey-Bass Publishers, San Francisco.

MacKinnon, R.J., Pukk-Härenstam, K., Kennedy, C., Hollnagel, E., Slater, D., 2021. A novel approach to explore Safety-I and Safety-II perspectives in in situ simulations-the structured what if functional resonance analysis methodology. Adv. Simul. (Lond). 6 (1), 21.

Management of Health and Safety at Work Regulations, 1999. https://www.legislation.gov.uk/uksi/1999/3242/contents/made.

National Health Service England, 2021. Patient Safety Incident Response Framework. https://www.england.nhs.uk/patient-safety/incident-response-framework/.

National Health Service Improvement, 2021. Framework for Involving Patients in Patient Safety. NHS Improvement, London.

National Health Service Improvement, 2018. Never Events Policy and Framework. NHS Improvement, London.

CHAPTER 4

Human Factors in Urgent, Unscheduled and Emergency Care

Anthony Kitchener

CHAPTER AIMS

1. Consider how human factors affect the approach paramedics take in caring for patients
2. Review the effects human factors have on patient care as part of the health system
3. Explore how differing agendas affect the approach of the paramedics
4. Examine the vectors of risk and how they link human factors to performance

Introduction

The out-of-hospital care provided by paramedics, ambulance crew and wider ambulance service provisions cover a spectrum of emergency, urgent, unscheduled and routine calls. This is illustrated in Fig. 4.1.

In the United Kingdom, in 2019–20, there were 12.4 million contacts to ambulance emergency operations centres, with 9.2 million coming from the general public. Of these 8.8 million were resolved either face-to-face or by 'hear and treat' over the telephone; 1.83 million were transferred to the ambulance service from the National Health Service (NHS); and 728,289 were referred by other healthcare professionals, such as general practitioners (AACE, 2021). There exist multiple system partners including NHS Hospital trusts, NHS community trusts, private ambulance services (PAS), voluntary/auxiliary ambulance partners, and multiple other healthcare organisations that contribute to or support the wider patient journey. Care undertaken in hospital settings involves a number of variables which are constants, such as work location, environmental factors and the ability to control the flow of people and access to different work areas (Holden et al., 2013). Conversely, when responding to 999 calls, stability and predictability are less certain. Mistakes related to human factors are often associated with environments and practices that are new or unfamiliar; therefore, out-of-hospital care is aligned with a high potential for human factor errors.

The use of the 999 ambulance service has evolved over the years and its contemporaneous workload far exceeds the transport service function that was the focus at its conception. In contemporary paramedic and ambulance practices, the focus is currently on the first contact practitioner role with the ambulance crew expected to be proficient in broad ranges of assessment, management and care planning aligned with a generalist portfolio. No longer is ambulance service care focussed just on emergency life or limb threatening presentations or significant accidents, although this is still part of the wider capabilities. Nowadays service extends across a spectrum of presentations including urgent and unscheduled care needs—adding to the level of complexities that make-up modern-day ambulance service. The professionalisation journey of the paramedic profession including the evolution of paramedic education has also allowed for more complex critical thinking, more automaticity in roles and a wider range of care options for any given situation (Brooks et al., 2016). In situations involving human factors, chances of human errors increase as the complexity evolves.

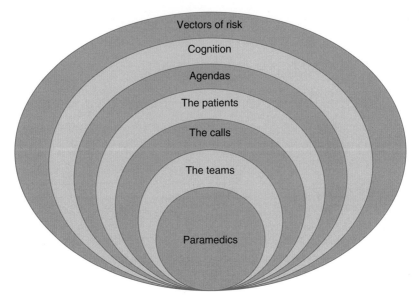

Fig. 4.1   Components of unscheduled, urgent emergency care.

TABLE 4.1 ■ **Examples of Job Roles Used in UK Ambulance Services**

Registered Healthcare Professionals	Nonregistered Healthcare Workers
Ambulance Nurse	Ambulance Technician
Newly Qualified Paramedic	Community First Responder
Paramedic	Emergency Care Support Worker
Senior Paramedic	Emergency Ambulance Crew
Clinical Team Mentors	Emergency Care Assistant
Clinical Supervisors	Apprentice Emergency Medical Technicians
Clinical/Paramedic Team Leaders	Emergency Medical Technicians 1, 2, 3
Managers/Leading Paramedics	Student Ambulance Paramedic 1, 2
Community Paramedics	Ambulance Technician
Emergency Care Practitioners	Apprentice Emergency Medical Technician
Specialist Paramedics	(supervised)
Advanced Paramedics	Associate Ambulance Practitioner
Advanced Clinical Practitioners	Senior Emergency Medical Technician
Consultant Paramedics	

Teams

The out-of-hospital care teams are made up of two core groups of people. The first group comprises registered healthcare professionals—their services correspond with the public's perception of the ambulance service. In the United Kingdom, paramedics are registered healthcare professionals regulated by the Health and Care Professions Council. The second group comprises those who work within the same clinical environment and are nonregistered healthcare workers, including emergency medical technicians (EMTs) and emergency care support workers (ECSWs). The inclusion of public as well as colleagues who work alongside these healthcare staff introduces scope for error when there is a lack of clarity regarding roles or their related competency. This related competency may be referred to as scope of practice. In general, it would be anticipated that with just two groups to consider the complexity is fairly shallow. When exploring the variations within these groups, there are extensive job roles and sub-scopes of practice, and there is no uniformed naming convention across the United Kingdom. Table 4.1 presents some examples of the variations in commonly used job roles, each of which have a differing set of knowledge, skills, behaviours and attributes. In case of an emergency or when a group of staff are brought together to respond to a call (who may have never met before), the complexity or roles and differing titles make errors ever more possible.

To further complicate situations, the ambulance service has a history of being a uniformed organisation with hierarchical rank structures. If there was a constant correlation with heightened rank against clinical capability, then this may be less confusing; however, rank and clinical ability are separate entities. You may have a senior ranked officer with a junior clinical qualification or a senior clinical qualification, above that of a colleague with them being a technical subordinate (e.g. paramedic team leaders are higher in rank but may not be necessarily as skilled as a paramedic). Some services have moved away from use of rank altogether to role identification in order to reduce misunderstandings and conflict of concepts. Some have taken this excessively far and have every job role title detailed on epaulettes. Some have a safe middle ground of ensuring the clinical grade is clearly identified on epaulettes and coat badges. Some services have further promoted a better human factors culture by using coloured epaulettes to denote specialism or status of a registered healthcare professional (Case Study 4.1).

CASE STUDY 4.1

You are a paramedic in a rapid response vehicle attending a life-threatening cardiac presentation and your patient may become unstable in the near future. You are rapidly backed up by a double-staffed ambulance with two crew members who are not clearly identified, and one is wearing one pip on their shoulder. The crew are out of area, so you have never met them before, and time is of the essence. If you, the paramedic, hand over the patientcare, but the crew does not have the scope of practice to effectively care for the patient, could the patient come to harm because of this lack of clarity about identification?

ATTITUDES AND BEHAVIOURS

Concepts of emotional labour, psychological safety and psychosocial resilience are linked to how we cope when working in healthcare (Williams and Kemp, 2019). Notwithstanding the diverse range of scope of practice and associated technical skills, ambulance staff come together to care for patients on multiple occasions. Often, those that work similar shift patterns will work alongside familiar colleagues and those who work mainly on rapid response vehicles will be backed-up by familiar colleagues working on double staffed ambulances. Where there is familiarity, human factors are supported by knowing how you and your colleagues tend to work. You will be familiar with phrasing, tone of voice, urgency of approach and general confidence levels in various presentations. Conversely, there is opportunity for conflict of opinions, clash of personalities and interactions of various behaviours which do not comfortably sit with your own ethical or moral stances. How an individual deals with these adverse challenges or clashes often reflects their own resilience and attitudes.

Picking a battle may, in the short term, provide individual gains; however, in the long term, this may compromise working relations or may even bring in doubt, pre-emptive defensiveness or nervousness about future interactions with colleagues. Future behaviours routed in previous interactions or even the reputation of previous connections could inadvertently affect the way you would otherwise advocate or care for your patient. This may make you hesitant to speak up when an incident may occur or inhibit you to challenge a practice which may not be optimal at that time. In this case, civility can often save lives and having professional civility in your interactions with colleagues at all times may prevent issues such as these from ever occurring (Case Study 4.2).

CASE STUDY 4.2

You attend a patient in cardiac arrest, the environment is pressured and appears chaotic. Your colleague 'snaps' at you to get on and perform chest compressions and berates you for your technique in front of a student you are mentoring. The patient had a successful outcome and was transported. You back-up the same colleague for another case a few hours later; you find yourself 'on edge' and therefore alter your behaviour to accommodate. As you do not approach the new patient in the same way you normally would, you make a mistake.

WORKING OUT OF AREA

Familiarity of area is often helpful and ambulance crews will become familiar with local 'hotspots' of activity. Common locations for calls include public houses, shopping centres, care homes, refuges and houses of frequent service users. The local crew will also be familiar with local care pathways which will allow patients to be cared for in the optimal way. Attendance at calls is digitised; from the moment of call connection, with details passed down to an electronic data terminal in a response vehicle or ambulance, this auto-programmes a satellite navigation system. Navigation systems are largely reliable; however, they have been known for suggesting routes across areas which are impassable or with prohibitive bollards that prevent access. Blindly following technology without local knowledge of these variations can waste precious time in responding to critically ill patients. Ambulance services are regionalised and work on a predictive algorithm to try and predict where the next resource is required; however, at peak demand, a dispatch may involve a crew travelling large distances and entering into unfamiliar territory. This could extend to not knowing the local healthcare pathways or becoming fully reliant upon technology to secure knowledge about how to complete a patient care journey (Case Study 4.3).

CASE STUDY 4.3

A crew is working a Friday night shift and has completed three previous calls, discharging each one on scene. With each of these calls, they have moved further and further out of area and are now over 60 miles away from their base station. The final call is 5 miles further away and the patient requires admission to the closest hyper-acute stroke unit. As a crew you are not sure of the closest hospital or which services it offers, so you must spend time looking this up and delaying patient transport time; the patient has long-term neurovascular damage due to the prolonged-on scene times.

CHOOSING CALL PRIORITY

Models of human behaviour such as the nature and patterns of human error, information processing, decision-making and teamwork have clear applications in healthcare. Human factors focus on a system view of safety, and propose that safety should, where possible, be 'designed in' (Norris, 2009). The 999-call system has a series of roles to ensure that someone ringing 999 for help has their call answered almost immediately. This role is normally undertaken by a nonclinical call handler. To prevent human error in these initial triage phases, a computer-based algorithm is followed which leads to call disposition (call categorisation). This removes the likelihood of human error in early data gathering. The use of a nonclinically trained call handler in the early stages removes the over thinking of any given presentation and priority. A decision about resource allocation is then made after categorisation and there are a number of options which could occur—some automated and some reliant upon the decision-making process of a call dispatcher or specialist teams within the ambulance control centre.

Automatic dispositions for lower acuity calls will go to a 'hear and treat' allocation where the patient will have a clinical assessment over the phone, but this may not be immediate. Telephone assessment is intrinsically higher risk given that physical assessment and visual assessment is not often available, and the care plan is based on a verbal history taking process (Vaona et al., 2001). These calls are undertaken by healthcare professionals typically including paramedics and nurses and are reliant upon the comprehensive interrogation of any given presenting case to decide an outcome or appropriate clinical advice. There is scope for human error in the gathering of this clinical information, risk stratification and outcome decisions. Often there is a queue of patients for this clinical triage care process, and the impact of knowing that others are waiting may alter the approach to a call and differ when system pressures are lower.

Having effective leadership to support decision making is key (Mercer et al., 2015). Critical care presentations may be allocated to a critical care desk to assess the requirement for advanced critical care interventions. These resources may include dispatch of local doctor schemes, dispatch of NHS Advanced Paramedics in Critical Care or mobilisation of Helicopter Emergency Medical Services (HEMS). These expert resources are often restricted where they are geographically dispersed and restricted due to triage allocation. Thus, when multiple calls come in, the decision made by a person as to which case may benefit from this specialist intervention may cause one patient being allocated this resource and another not receiving this enhanced care. This human factor risk is often mitigated by having an experienced critical care practitioner make the decision, thus aligning their scope of practice to hone the need or likely impact any team intervention.

Another team with a similar level of complexity and allocation is the Hazardous Area Response Team (HART). HART specialist practitioners deal with urban search and rescue, water rescue, mass casualty incidents, complex rescues and terrorist related incidents. This highly specialist resource is often extremely geographically dispersed with maybe one or two HART teams across an entire NHS trust; again, the allocation decision will alter the course of such a significant incident.

In the same stream of thinking, advanced practitioners in urgent and primary care and dispatchers of community first responders and specific scheme cars (such as those for mental health response, occupational therapy falls, prehospital care doctors) are all reliant on individual dispatch decisions at any given time and are balanced against the overall call demands. The ambulance control centre can have conflicting pressures, periods of high demand and a rationing of resources when call volume outweighs the ability to respond until call demand reduces. As resources deplete, allocation decisions weigh much more heavily on individual choice—thus, the human factor risk is heightened (Case Study 4.4).

CASE STUDY 4.4

It is late evening on a paid bank-holiday day and there is heightened demand across all areas. Three simultaneous emergency calls come in for a stabbing, a fall from height and a road traffic collision with reported fatalities. There is one local enhanced care service available for dispatch and the critical care desk allocated it to the victim of the stabbing. The other two emergencies did not benefit from enhanced care.

TABLE 4.2 ■ Human Factors Which May Inhibit Patient–Practitioner Communication

Transmission of Out-of-Hospital Communication	Receiving of Out-of-Hospital Communication
Access to the patient	Strength of phone signal/reception
Health agenda of any caller	Clarity of received answers
Patient age	Active listening
Learning difficulties or disabilities	Understanding what has been said
Foreign language speaker	Interpretation of what has been said
Patient anxiety or mental health	Previous interactions with the patient
Pain levels	Tiredness of the clinician
Delusional states	Bandwidth of the clinician
Reduced levels of consciousness	
Cognitive impairment from alcohol	
Expressive aphasia or dysphonia	
Influence of other people around	
Being in a public place	
Surround/background noise	

PATIENTS AND HISTORY

There are various examples of where human factors exist within the prehospital profession. Common examples are environmental distractions including noise from bystanders, mobile phones, machines, lack of sleep and inadequate nourishment (Summers and Willis, 2013). Paramedics are familiar with taking patient history and communication is key to building a comprehensive clinical picture on which to base an outcome decision. There are several factors which may inhibit the ability to effectively communicate. Communication can be divided into the two elements of transmission and receiving. Table 4.2 presents some examples of human factors that may inhibit effective communication.

Patient presentations are often complex and built on an evolving picture of healthcare. The ability of a practitioner to ask appropriate questions, receive, interpret and weigh up the relevance of any given information is a complex area and reflects the need for extensive education in patient assessment techniques. Paraphrasing and clarification of patient answers is often helpful and exploring particular points of unclarity again can support obtaining relevant information on which to base an out-of-hospital care plan. In prehospital care training, there is a particular lean towards excluding life-threatening presentation and the use of a 'red flag' approach, which includes questions that imply a more sinister pathological underlying presentation, is often helpful but may be less holistic in approach. This dichotomy of urgent interrogation to evaluate life or limb threatening presentations and implement rapid treatment decision is balanced against the time it takes to comprehensively undertake a full medical clerking process. It relies on human interpretation of the system; reactive decision to determine urgency; and what, if any, elements of a clinical work-up should be left to focus on rapid treatment instead.

An example is the 10 minutes on scene approach for identifying acute prehospital stroke presentations, which aims to reduce on scene time to less than 10 minutes for hyper acute strokes. If this is applied correctly, it can improve outcome survivability of stroke presentations; conversely, wider and more holistic considerations of care may be overlooked or not considered. The approach taken to gain the minimal set of information on which to make a safe and rapid decision will rely on the ability of the respective clinicians to prioritise questioning and interpret the data presented to them. What is it about the environment that may inhibit every clinician for every stroke case from making this happen? Examples may include the inability to gain effective history via communication techniques, concerns about welfare for pets on scene and difficulties in securing the property, in addition to any number of variable factors which may inhibit the clear compliance to this approach.

It is important to not only activate rapid treatment pathways where appropriate, but also exclude those who should not be accessing these—thus not 'clogging' the system with false positives which may detrimentally affect access for another patient to that system at similar times. It is often difficult for an individual who is so close to the scene and entangled in the patient presentation to consider the broader system-wide impact beyond that of the individual patient (the conflict of here and now).

LENS OF AGENDA

Front-line ambulance staff often make decisions that are time critical and based on limited information, but wrong decisions in this context can have serious consequences for patients (O'Hara et al., 2014). Being aware of respective agendas can be difficult, in that the patient may have different ideas, concerns or expectations related to their own health, which could even extend to health anxieties. They may be cognisant of how busy the ambulance service or receiving hospitals are and may try and influence your decisions by providing information that suits their respective agenda. This may be different to the pure pathological information and can be shaped by a vast range of individual backgrounds. As a clinician you will be educated in appraising medical presentations and correlating the symptoms for a likely diagnosis; however, sometimes things just do not add up. Frustrations may creep in, and this may affect professional evaluation of a given situation, when a better understanding of the patient agenda may actually balance the human instinct for mistrust.

Conversely, the system pressures clinicians to perform in certain ways. Clinical effectiveness is measured against performance targets and care bundles (groups of assessment or treatments audited for compliance). There is also a culture around risk appetite and whether it is safer to transfer the patient to a hospital for a more senior opinion. It is questionable whether these external factors influence the way we care for patients and whether the 'health agenda' pushes a patient care journey in a certain direction and changes the way we may behave as healthcare professionals (Case Study 4.5). After all, who are you treating, the patient or the audit bundle?

CASE STUDY 4.5

You are called out to a 74-year-old man who is presenting with a chest infection and you think he has sepsis. You are keen to treat the patient as per the sepsis care bundle and rapid transport to the hospital. The patient does not want to go to hospital and decides that he just wants to stay at home. The crew respect his wishes and leave. On exiting the property, the crew meet his daughter who mentions that his wife Elsie was admitted to hospital and died from pneumonia. Knowing this information could have changed the approach for dealing with this patient because the patient had an agenda of not going to the place where his wife died.

BANDWIDTH

There are a number of occupational stresses experienced by paramedics and ambulance crews (Mahony, 2001). Out-of-hospital care situations can be complex environments (Summers and Willis, 2010). It is questionable how complicated an environment becomes before the cognitive bandwidths of the respective clinicians on scene become overwhelmed. Imagine you are called to a cardiac arrest, a common presentation with which paramedic crews are familiar. Now imagine

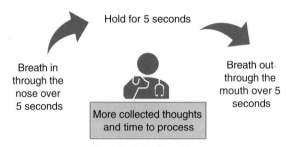

Fig. 4.2 Active breathing.

that patient is trapped in a car on a busy main road. Add to this the following scenarios: there are three other people in the car, two of which are screaming children in the back; it is nighttime and very cold; the paramedic has been busy all night and is feeling very tired; and the paramedic has been having issues at home, is worried about relationship issues, is late in finishing and has been thinking about this on the way to the call. At what point does cognitive bandwidth becomes compromised and the ability to make decisions becomes less optimal?

There are several methods used to overcome complexities involving repetitive simulation training and the use of muscle memory to undertake safe approaches. These skill drills, repeated over and over again, will lead a paramedic to undertake a more automatic approach to care. The back-to-basics approach is often used and mnemonics such as the A–E (airway, breathing, circulation, disability, exposure) approach is a steadfast guide for getting through a complex situation even when it seems overwhelming. The amount of information or bandwidth needed to complete a process a complex task can be challenging (Grootjen et al., 2006). Breathing cycles is a useful method that gives you a few moments time to think and process (the 15-second approach to care) and active breathing (Fig. 4.2) may supress the adrenaline response and allow you to scan the scene to support the input of the complex information.

Top Tip: The 15-second approach to care is a short cycle of breathing used when faced with a potentially overwhelming bandwidth situation, giving a short pause to absorb and process. It involves breathing through the nose for 5 seconds, holding for 5 seconds and breathing out through the mouth over 5 seconds. This process can help suppress the adrenaline response which will keep you feel calmer. You can use this time to look around, and these seconds may help you manage a situation much more effectively.

Equipment Familiarity

Ambulance service personnel face a disproportionally high risk for fatality and injury due to the nature of their work (Du et al., 2019). Part of the out-of-hospital assessment and treatment involves using ambulance equipment. Adverse events may occur during ambulance equipment operation and result in significant injury to patients and ambulance personnel (Wang et al., 2009). Preparing the equipment and a daily vehicle inspection ahead of responding to make sure you have everything that you will need is important. In high pressure ambulance systems, there are often calls outstanding and waiting for ambulance response that may result in mobilisation before full checks can be carried out. There is a risk that due to lack of preparations individual performance may be compromised further down the line. This underpins the need for allotted time at the start of a shift prior to dispatch for safety checks and equipment preparation prior.

Familiarity with equipment can be an area where the individual may fall short in proficiency; however, having a standard layout may reduce human factor errors (Yuval et al., 2015). For example, if you are proficient with one particular type of cardiac monitor and have used it multiple times, you will be confident with this piece of equipment. Imagine though that you are sent across county borders to back up a colleague from a neighbour ambulance service and they are using a different monitor. The patient deteriorates and you are asked to perform urgent cardiac electro-cardiogram (ECG) and you are not clear on how to use it. In normal circumstances you would be highly proficient in this process, but due to the equipment change your competency is reduced. Further, complexity of equipment may affect the ability of the user to safely use it (Ferreira and Hignett, 2005); for example, equipment that is not used routinely may lead to reduced proficiency (Case Study 4.6).

CASE STUDY 4.6

You are called to a patient who has been kicked in the upper thigh by a horse. The upper leg has a barrel shape to it. You diagnose a mid-shaft femur fracture and want to apply a traction splint. You have not used a traction splint for over 2 years and are unfamiliar with its application. You manage to apply the splint, but incorrectly, and it does not traction the leg properly—meaning treatment is ineffective.

To reduce skill knowledge attrition and promote competency, despite nonregular use, equipment can be made more human factor friendly. Simplicity in design with logically flowing processes can often be helpful. This has been observed in the use of commercial computers, tablets and mobile telephones. Intuitive process are often meaningful, as even when users have had no experience with such a device, they can rapidly learn to use it.

RISK VECTORS

Human factors are a spectrum of possibilities and in out-of-hospital care these can be aligned with various risk vectors. The severity of illness (very sick vs a little sick) approach affects how we interpret and process information. In extreme situations and with repetitive exposures to low acuity presentations, this may lead to false confidence or underestimations of healthcare presentations. In the extremes for acuity, the focus of care becomes narrowed and associated rapidity can mean haste in the assessment technique. This is balanced against the vector of familiarity. When a crew is familiar with a presentation, their competency and approach become much more effective. Paramedics will regularly assess patients who have fallen, with chest pains and who are short of breath. When presentation is more rare or unfamiliar, the ability to make mistakes are heightened. Differing crews will have different experiences; therefore, individual variations are difficult to plan for when the presentation is rare (Case Study 4.7).

CASE STUDY 4.7

A crew is called out to an 18-year-old who has new onset diarrhoea and vomiting. They have a background of juvenile arthritis which is being treated by a disease modifying anti-heumatic drug. This drug makes the patient immunosuppressed. The crew are unfamiliar with this treatment process for the musculoskeletal condition and do not take this into account with the management plan. They advise the patient to self-treat for gastroenteritis. Two hours after discharge the patient deteriorates into life threatening sepsis.

The attending crew may also deal with an incident in different ways depending on their competency. If they are relatively novice in their clinical practice, their knowledge, skills, behaviours and other attributes may cause different responses to a challenging situation than those with expert clinical practice. Similarly, when paramedics have advanced clinical practice, their aligned specialties may enhance their abilities to deal with a situation. At any given time, the position along the vector can change and the position can be influenced by external factors (Fig. 4.3).

Therefore, the outcome is that performance in the out-of-hospital care environment can be positioned, and when awareness of this exists it can be manipulated to reduce the influence of human factors. People undertaking a performance task will operate at one of four levels, with the workload being optimal, underloaded, overloaded or vigilant (Grootjen et al., 2006). Organisational factors such as low job autonomy, lack of supervisor support and poor leadership are impacting the health and well-being of frontline ambulance workers (Harrison, 2019) and may be linked to the vectors described.

Overconfidence is an identified human factor in the out-of-hospital care sector. Compared to other areas of community and hospital-based healthcare, there is no other professional group with such a spectrum of autonomous practice with relatively comparative junior clinical grades. This combined with the isolation factor can lead to a cyclical reinforcement, indicating that practice is never challenged or adapted (Fig. 4.4).

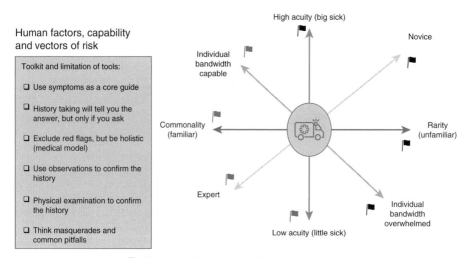

Fig. 4.3   Human factors, capability and risk vectors.

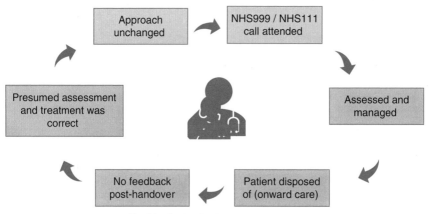

Fig. 4.4   Cycle of uniformed persistency.

WHEN THINGS GO WRONG

Out-of-hospital emergencies are often managed by a team of people from the ambulance service, which as previously described can be made up of registered healthcare professionals and nonregistered healthcare workers. Nonclinical skills are required to achieve management in an information-poor environment and minimise the risk of errors (Bleetman et al., 2012). There is legal responsibility to be honest when things go wrong; this is also reflected through the need for honest conduct and professional integrity incumbent of people working in a public office. Things that can go wrong are highlighted by complaints and significant incident reports being filed. They can also be highlighted by crew at the scene or individuals involved in patient care later on in the care journey path, such as by hospital colleagues.

The ambulance service has a clear clinical and organisational hierarchy that may inhibit people from speaking up and when crews have not worked together before, a lack of familiarity may add to these barriers. Effective teamwork is desirable to improve patient outcomes (Miller, 2015). Simple steps can be taken to overcome this, including providing opportunities for colleagues to speak up and having a defined leader who can step back and keep a high-level view rather than be in the focussed work area (Fig. 4.5).

Having defined roles can help reduce the opportunity for human error (Salas et al., 2007), but unlike in a hospital there may not be an optimal number of teams on scene. For example, you are working solo on a rapid response call. All the roles are yours until a bigger team arrives and establishes themselves, and a leader emerges depending upon who arrives and their respective backgrounds (Tuckman, 1965). While you are operating multiple roles, the likelihood for mistakes may be higher. Conversely, all information and ownership sit with you, so the control of information and need for communication is lessened. Communication is key, the best practice to do a 'round of introductions' as each new team member is added including name and skills grade for absolute clarity. Using names in a busy environment will also prevent misunderstanding and allow individuals to respond to any challenges directed at them. When given a specific task, such as leading for the airway, a crew member may become 'in the zone' and their peripheral awareness reduces as they focus on the task at hand. It is vital that all team members respond, and using their names can be helpful if this is not certain. With the possibility of sharp injuries or accidental defibrillation of a crew member, their health and safety are dependent on effective communication.

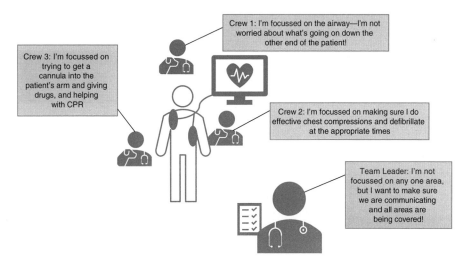

Fig. 4.5 Focussed vs overview.

PRACTICE MAKES PERFECT

In the complexities of an emergency, there are a number of ways reliance on individual memory or complex decision making can be planned out. Utilising pocketbooks or digital apps which can give you precise details is an ideal approach. For example, undertaking complex paediatric calculations—if you were faced with a paediatric drowning and had to administer intravenous adrenaline, you would not want to be undertaking extended calculations to get the right dose; instead, it is preferable to avoid the chance of human error by checking it against a pre-calculated figure. This could be further extended to all elements of drug administration including indications, contraindications, side effects and cautions. The habitual use of checking and using checklists to ensure that human error is reduced is an underused approach in the out-of-hospital care settings (Marshall and Touzell, 2020).

Top Tip: If in doubt, check it out [clinical guidelines]

Skill drills are a way of reinforcing muscle memory; regularly practicing psycho-motor skills reduces the chance of human error for skills that are infrequently used, perfects these skills, and avoids skill fade. There are numerous skills that paramedics use to alter the course of life-threatening pathologies. Needle cricothyroidotomy and needle thoracocentesis are two interventions that paramedics may need to make; however, they can be extremely rare. Some paramedics will never use these skills on an actual patient during their entire career and others may use them once in a year. In situations where implementing these skills could be the difference between life or death, not being proficient in implementing immediate intervention may compromise capability. Practice, experience and for example simulation training can help mitigate errors and hesitation due to lack of experience but can vary from one clinician to the next.

Conclusion

This chapter demonstrated the centrality and understanding of human factors in a complex system where unpredictability and risks are constant. Being skilled and competent is a good start, but safe care is also reliant on teamwork, a joined-up approach of the different parts (from the frontline to the call centre) and a smooth functioning system. Nontechnical skills combined with technical skills are not only crucial for safe care but can fundamentally help reduce errors in communication, drug administration and misdiagnosis. Additionally, responders must learn to manage multiple stressors, lead in difficult circumstances and manage the tasks and team to sustain performance successfully.

References

AACE, 2021. Annual Report 2019-2020. Association of Ambulance Chief Executives, London.

Bleetman, A., Sanusi, S., Dale, T., Brace, S., 2012. Human factors and error prevention in emergency medicine. Emerg. Med. J. 29 (5), 389–393.

Brooks, I.A., Cooke, M., Spencer, C., Archer, F., 2016. A review of key national reports to describe the development of paramedic education in England (1966–2014). Emerg. Med. J. 33 (12), 876–881.

Du, B., Boileau, M., Wierts, K., Hignett, S., Fischer, S., Yazdani, A., 2019. Existing science on human factors and ergonomics in the design of ambulances and EMS equipment. Prehosp. Emerg. Care 23 (5), 103–267.

Ferreira, J., Hignett, S., 2005. Reviewing ambulance design for clinical efficiency and paramedic safety. Appl. Ergon. 36 (1), 97–105.

Grootjen, M., Neerincx, M., Veltman, J.A., 2006. Cognitive task load in a naval ship control centre: from identification to prediction. Ergonomics 49 (12–13), 1238–1264.

Harrison, J., 2019. Organisational factors: impacting on health for ambulance personnel. Int. J. Emerg. Serv. 8 (2), 134–146.

Holden, R.J., Carayon, P., Gurses, A.P., Hoonakker, P., Hundt, A.S., Ozok, A.A., et al., 2013. Seips 2.0: a human factors framework for studying and improving the work of healthcare professionals and patients. Ergonomics 56 (11), 1669–1686.

Mahony, K.L., 2001. Management and the creation of occupational stressors in an Australian and a UK Ambulance Service. Aust. Health Rev. 24 (4), 135–145.

Marshall, S.D., Touzell, A., 2020. Human factors and the safety of surgical and anaesthetic care. Anaesthesia 75 (Suppl. 1), e34–e38.

Mercer, S., Park, C., Tarmey, N.T., 2015. Human factors in complex trauma. BJA Educ. 15 (5), 231–236.

Miller, J., 2015. Better together? ambulance staff views of human factors in resuscitation. Emerg. Med. J. 32 (6), e14.

Norris, B., 2009. Human factors and safe patient care. Nurs. Manag. 17 (2), 203–211.

O'Hara, R., Johnson, M., Hirst, E., Weyman, A., Shaw, D., Mortimer, P., et al., 2014. A Qualitative Study of Decision-Making and Safety in Ambulance Service Transitions. NIHR Journals Library, Southampton (UK).

Salas, E., Rosen, M.A., King, H.B., 2007. Managing teams managing crises: principles of teamwork to improve patient safety in the emergency room and beyond. Theor. Issues Ergon. Sci. 8 (5), 381–394.

Summers, A., Willis, S., 2010. Human factors within paramedic practice: the forgotten paradigm. J. Paramedic Pract. 2 (9), 424–428.

Summers, A., Willis, S., 2013. Human factors within paramedic practice: the forgotten paradigm. J. Paramedic Pract. 2 (9), 1759 –1376.

Tuckman, B.W., 1965. Developmental sequence in small groups. Psychol. Bull. 63, 384–399.

Vaona, A., Pappas, Y., Grewal, R.S., Ajaz, M., Majeed, A., Car, J., 2001. Training interventions for improving telephone consultation skills in clinicians. Cochrane Database Syst. Rev. 1 (1), CD010034.

Wang, H.E., Weaver, M.D., Abo, B.N., Kaliappan, R., Fairbanks, R.J., 2009. Ambulance stretcher adverse events. Qual. Saf. Health Care 18 (3), 213–216.

Williams, R., Kemp, V., 2019. Caring for healthcare practitioners. BJPsych Adv. 26, 116–128.

Yuval, B., Ramey, S., Giselle, P., Tarmo, V., 2015. Working with paramedics on implementing human factors improvements to their response bags. Proc. Int. Symp. Hum. Factors Ergon. Healthc. 4 (1), 179–181.

Nontechnical Skills

Zubeir Essat

1. Understand the impact of human factors and nontechnical skills on patient safety
2. Understand how nontechnical skills are assessed in practice
3. Consider the validity, reliability and practicality of these assessments
4. Understand challenges faced when assessing nontechnical skills in pre and post registered nurses and allied healthcare professionals. The focus is on nursing practice, but this chapter is applicable to all allied healthcare practices
5. Discuss how we can increase nontechnical skills awareness, advance a nontechnical skills profile in healthcare education and suggest strategies to incorporate nontechnical and human factors in health education

Introduction

Nontechnical skills belong to the realm of a wider skillset related to human factors. Human factors encompass aspects not only individual characteristics but also environmental and institutional aspects that impact performance and safety (White, 2012). Nontechnical skills comprise social, cognitive and personal resource skills that affect individual and small team performances (Flin et al., 2008). Social skills include communication, leadership and followership. Cognitive skills include task allocation, fixation, setting priorities and planning. Personal resource skills include strategies to cope with stress, fatigue and resilience.

It has long been demonstrated that lack of technical skills and knowledge do not always lead to medical errors but rather a failure to understand and appreciate the effects of nontechnical skills on safety.

This chapter will explore the impact of human factors in the healthcare arena with a focus on how patient safety is affected, and how nontechnical skills are assessed in the pre and post curricula of nurses, midwifes and allied health professionals.

There are many challenges in raising the profile of nontechnical skills in healthcare. This chapter shares some strategies to aid your practice and that are aimed to be incorporated in healthcare education in academic and practice settings.

Case Study

Nontechnical skills were clearly demonstrated in the failure to respond appropriately in a medical emergency surrounding the case involving Mrs Bromiley. You can view this case study reconstruction online, titled *Just a Routine Operation* (https://www.youtube.com/watch?v=JzlvgtPIof4). This case study focuses on a patient, Mrs. Bromiley, who had been admitted for nasal surgery. While anaesthetising Mrs. Bromiley, the anaesthetist lost the airway and could not insert an endotracheal tube or a laryngeal mask. Another anaesthetist and an ear nose and throat (ENT) surgeon entered the room to help and despite several attempts to intubate the patient and administer drugs to relax the airway, all three experienced doctors could not intubate the patient. The patient was experiencing a medical emergency called 'can't oxygenate can't intubate'. There was a care pathway and protocol for this emergency; however, it was not consulted and not as robustly applied as in contemporary plans.

An emergency tracheostomy and level three acute care bed would have helped in this emergency. However, the three experienced doctors did not choose these options; instead, they decided to stop the procedure and allowed Mrs. Bromiley to wake up naturally in the recovery room. During this 40-minute emergency episode, Mrs. Bromiley's oxygen saturation level was very low—as low as 40% for minutes. This led to hypoxic brain injury; Mrs. Bromiley never regained consciousness and, sadly, she subsequently died a few days later in intensive care.

QUESTIONS

What went wrong in this case? Why did the doctors not insert an emergency tracheostomy as they should have? Why did they persevere with a plan to intubate that was clearly not working? Why did they not stop and oxygenate the patient? Why did they not realise the oxygen saturation level was low? Why did they ignore the nonmedical staff about the intensive therapy unit (ITU) bed? Why did the alarms on the monitor not trigger their attention? What we can conclude is that the issue was not lack of experience or qualifications of the medical staff involved. Considering that these anaesthetists and surgeon had years of experience and were senior staff members, why did they act the way they did?

These questions can be applied to numerous other clinical incidences; however, they are seldom analysed and retained for lessons learnt. We tend to focus on the negative aspects of incidences and do not always highlight good practices or exemplary efforts which inadvertently improve patient safety.

ANALYSIS

If we look at the case in more detail, the nursing staff did recognise the 'can't ventilate can't intubate' medical emergency, brought a tracheostomy surgical tray and booked an intensive care bed. Regrettably, the doctors did not act upon the tray being delivered and did not perform a tracheostomy. The medical team also thought that an ITU bed was not necessary, and thus one of the nurses cancelled the bed booking. Therefore, the root cause was not a lack of technical expertise but failures in nontechnical skills.

One of these failures revolves around situational awareness. The medical team simply lost track of time (White, 2012); they got fixated in inserting the endotracheal tube to such an extent that they were blinded to other options. They became so absorbed in this procedure that they could not see the bigger picture; they did not step back and consult with the nursing team (e.g. 'Look we have tried intubating a couple of times and it is not working. Has anyone got thoughts or other options?'). This important form of communication technique called a 'huddle', and would have allowed the team to step back and quickly consider what was happening, what was not working and what options were available to fix the situation. However, this did not happen and the nonappreciation of human factors in this case sadly contributed to the negative outcome. We will refer to this case later in this chapter.

> What can you say about the mental model of the team? Did they have the same mental image at the time?

When looking at the wider situation of safety failures in healthcare due to human factors, the figures are clear. Examinations of cases and research in healthcare errors worldwide show that a significant number of cases are attributable to human factors failures and they are the causes of death and serious injury to patients (Glavin and Maran, 2003; Merry, 2007; Morgan et al., 2009; Wauben et al., 2011; Westli et al., 2010; Zausig et al., 2009).

Therefore, it would be beneficial to teach nontechnical skills to nurses and allied healthcare practitioners and have their competency assessed. Unlike doctors who are exposed to simulation training in pre and postgraduation, these skills are rarely assessed for nursing or other healthcare professions unless they work in acute areas or perioperative practice. In preregistration curriculum, simulation training has only recently started to be considered as part of training (see Appendix 1 for simulation templates).

ASSESSMENT TOOLS

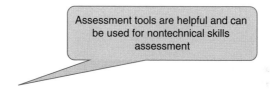

Assessment tools are helpful and can be used for nontechnical skills assessment

Other high-risk industries such as aviation, nuclear power and the military have long recognised the existence of human factors. In these industries, human factors and nontechnical skills competence is assessed in training and practice. It is not surprising that early examples of assessment tools for nontechnical skills were taken from these disciplines (Higham et al., 2019). Since then, several assessments have been developed for various settings and team usage in healthcare. Higham et al. (2019) found 76 competency assessment tools for nontechnical skills across healthcare, but if we just look at competency assessments which include other professionals such as nurses, the number is much smaller. Pires et al. (2017) found 16 assessment tools in the literature that include nurses and nursing teams. A summarised sample of six of these assessment tools is presented in Table 5.1 to show how these tools vary in content, setting, scoring, skills assessed, reliability and validity.

If we take a closer look at Table 5.1, we realise there is no general agreement as to which nontechnical skills are most significant. Each assessment tool assesses different nontechnical skills and, to a certain extent, different professionals. Some nontechnical skills, such as communication, are considered more important because they appear in multiple tools. However, depending on where you work, you will have to pick the most relevant assessment. In addition, the perception of which nontechnical skills are important can depend on which healthcare professional group you ask. A surgeon or anaesthetist may assume that 'assertiveness', being 'forthright and confident about having the best judgement' and 'being in control' in an acute emergency would be deemed important nontechnical skills. Anaesthetists and surgeons have their own validated nontechnical skills assessment tools, the anaesthetists' nontechnical skills (ANTS) and the nontechnical skills for surgeons (NOTTS) tools, respectively. However, nurses and allied health professionals may consider nontechnical skills such as 'humility' and 'admitting own fallibility' to be more important for surgeons or anaesthetists (Larsson, 2013; Stiglich, 2019).

The differences in the nontechnical skills being assessed is also partly because certain tools are to be used in specific settings or with specific teams or healthcare groups. Different settings will require different nontechnical skills to be assessed. Most tools tend to focus on acute care and are set mainly in operating theatres or emergency/intensive care environments (Higham, 2019). Therefore, these tools have a narrow scope of application. Areas such as mental health, community care and less acute areas of care have few assessment tools available.

> A generic nontechnical skills tools could be beneficial although components may vary. Generic competencies such as communication for a mental health nurse mayinclude verbal de-escalation techniques which other nurses working in different settings may need to know as well.

Future development of generic nursing orientated assessment tools would certainly go a long way to correct this disparity and be a valuable resource for developing nursing practice and increasing safety. Appendix 1 presents how nontechnical skills observation or assessment can be part of any clinical scenario and a crucial part of learning.

Another aspect of these assessment tools is that they are mainly concerned with patient safety and do not look specifically at other facets of nursing care such as efficiency and increased productivity. A misconception of nursing leaders is that improvement in patient safety and error reduction will improve quality of care and efficiency. Including these other facets in the tool could improve uptake of the nontechnical skills tools. If we compare how a formula one pit crew use repeated simulation to examine how the crew will react to possible different scenarios in a future race, we will see that the pit crew are not only reviewing performance safety but also performance efficiency. Some have argued that assessing skills that increase efficiency, reduce resource use and cost and increase patient experience and job role satisfaction will make the nontechnical skills tools more palatable. However, these can be discussed and elaborated upon in debriefs and huddles after simulation training.

How the tools are scored also varies; the scoring systems tend to have rating scores that vary in number and scale. Some tools have descriptors for good or poor demonstration of nontechnical skills whilst others use numerical values. Usability differs between tools; some require formal training while others are designed for ease of use and require little or no training. Regardless of whether training is recommended, training should be highly recommended for accuracy and reliability of results.

Observing nontechnical skills can be subtle and nuanced, and thus having experienced trainers can be of great benefit. However, offering training will invariably have financial and logistical implications. Training lectures and practice mentors would be costly and time consuming; although, it would confer huge benefits in terms of more reliable and accurate results. A way around this difficulty could be online training, which could introduce nontechnical skills and highlight the importance of understanding them in terms of patient safety.

Currently, the assessment tools available are most definitely useful when assessing nurses in acute care or within surgical teams and subsequently their use is recommended. Nurses, allied health professional tutors and nurse educators need to bear in mind the limitations inherent in these tools. If we take these tools seriously, as we should, the nursing profession needs to strive to create and develop assessment tools that are applicable for a wide variety of settings and focussed on nurses and nursing teams.

Thus far in this chapter, we have discussed why the assessment of nontechnical skills is important and how this has a direct impact on patient safety. We then discussed the assessment tools available to assess these skills. If we can agree that nontechnical skills are important, understanding them can help reduce patient harm and mortality and that these skills can be evaluated using the assessment tools available, our next question is how are we training nurses and other allied healthcare professionals to understand and develop these key skills?

Good common sense suggests that we will greatly improve patient safety by developing these skills both at the university undergraduate level and throughout postregistration careers.

TABLE 5.1 ■ Analysis of Nontechnical Skills Tools

Instruments	Assessment of Nontechnical Skills	Participants	Environment	Scoring	Reliability	Validity
Revised nontechnical skills (NOTECHS) (Sevdalis et al., 2008)	Communication/interaction; situational awareness/vigilance; cooperation/team skills; leadership; managerial	Scrub nurses, anaesthetists, surgeons, operating department practitioners	Simulated	Whole team; real time rating; 6-point rating scale	Internal consistency	Construct
Nontechnical skills in nurse anaesthetists (N-ANTS) (Lyk-Jensen et al., 2014)	Situational awareness; decision-making; task management; team working	Nurse anaesthetist	Simulated and real	Individual nurses; video playback rating; 5-point rating scale	Internal consistency; inter-rater	Content
Trauma nontechnical skills (t-NOTECHS) (Steinemann et al., 2012)	Communication/interaction; situation awareness/coping with stress; cooperation/resource; leadership; assessment/decision-making	Trauma/critical care nurse, trauma/critical care surgeons, trauma/medical intensivists	Simulated and real	Whole team; video playback rating; real time rating; 5-point rating scale	Internal consistency; inter-rater	Construct
Team emergency assessment measure (TEAM) (Cooper et al., 2010)	Leadership; teamwork; task management	Emergency resuscitation teams (nurses, student nurses, doctors, medical students)	Simulated and real	Whole team; video playback rating; real time rating; 5-point rating scale	Internal consistency; inter-rater; test-retest	Content; construct; unidimensional; concurrent
Scrub practitioners' list of intraoperative nontechnical skills (SPLINTS) (Mitchell et al., 2012)	Communication/teamwork; task management; situation awareness	Operating theatre scrub nurses and practitioners	Simulated and real	Individual nurses; video playback rating; 4-point rating scale	Inter-rater	Content
Ottawa Crisis Resource Management Global Rating Scale (Ottawa GRS) (Kim et al., 2006)	Problem-solving; situational awareness; leadership; resource utilisation; communication	All specialities of healthcare in acute care settings	Simulated	Individual nurse; video playback rating; point rating scale	Internal consistency; inter-rater	Construct

Adapted from Pires et al. (2017) and Higham et al. (2019).

Simulation use is an ideal way to teach and highlight the importance of nontechnical skills in relation to patient safety. Unlike in medicine, where nontechnical skills are assessed and addressed during mandatory simulation-based training for foundation and specialist training programmes, there is little or no provision for mandated simulation training in other health professions (Gjeraa et al., 2016; Peddle, 2015).

NONTECHNICAL SKILLS AND THE UNDERGRADUATE PROVISION

The complexities of healthcare provision have changed markedly over the last few decades. Increased specialisation, extended roles, greater use of technology and huge advances in medical science result in practitioners working in high-paced, high-risk environments that are physically and mentally demanding. In contrast, it can be argued that education programmes have not kept up with modern nursing practices. It is very important that our next generation of nurses are not underprepared and in danger of not being able to keep pace with role demands and workforce changes (Frenk et al., 2010). The perils of having nurse education curricula that does not tackle nontechnical skills and human factors are that patient safety can be compromised and put nurses at risk of being involved in healthcare errors that can have emotionally traumatic effects and potentially cause staff to leave the profession.

Therefore, what could be the reasons preventing simulation in pre and postregistration courses? Possible reasons are that educators and lecturers may be underprepared because their workload does not permit preparation time and the number of students in the programme render simulation unrealistic; these situations cannot be remedied unless substantial investments are made and educators are allowed to create and adapt. Some may view simulations as irrelevant, not yet fully understand what nontechnical skills are or assume that nontechnical skills will be developed through clinical experiences during placements and throughout clinical careers (Peddle, 2015; Peddle et al., 2020). However, there could also be reluctance to add simulation in the teaching programmes, especially when the programmes are already full and without spare teaching time. Another difficulty is that nursing courses have large numbers of students in each cohort. Delivering simulation sessions that will allow each student to participate in a meaningful way could become logistically difficult.

However, developing nontechnical skills does not necessarily require a simulation suite with a high-fidelity mannequin. Nontechnical skills can be taught using quizzes, games, objective structured clinical examinations (OCSEs) and virtual reality technology. The use of virtual reality technology is a potential answer to deliver simulations to large groups of students. Technology that utilises a virtual patient scenario, presented via a computer or mobile device in which the student has predetermined actions that need to be chosen to move the scenario along until a conclusion is reached, could be a valuable teaching tool. Thereby, we have a branching narrative; the student reaches a positive or negative outcome depending on the choices the made during the scenario (Peddle et al., 2020). Virtual scenarios can be completed at home as private study so they do not require timetabling or large groups of students and can be used for feedback and debriefing during class.

For educational establishments to commence using simulations, there needs to be a cultural shift for how educationists value simulations and recognise the importance of nontechnical skills. Once teaching space is allocated for simulations, educators need to decide on how to deliver the simulations. Ideally, educators would need to receive sufficient training in writing simulations so that learning outcomes can be achieved. Educationalists need training on how to deliver feedback and conduct debriefing sessions. Universities and colleges running healthcare courses must appreciate that the single most important aspect of any simulation is not how realistic or how high the fidelity is, but how skilfully feedback and debriefing is delivered. Debriefing is the single most important element; during the debriefing session is when the learning takes place (Jaye et al., 2015).

A successful simulation does not focus on whether the student made the right choices and treated the patient correctly without any errors, but rather on what the student needs to understand is why they acted the way they did. Making errors and getting it wrong is not the issue, it is the skill of the tutor to support the student, understand their thoughts and feeling during a simulation and observe what their thought processes were during each stage of the simulation. The students should be guided to explore their internal thought processes and become more self-aware of how they interpret the external environment, respond to a rapidly changing medical emergency, delegate and communicate to team members, prioritise actions and utilise the resources that are available to them. By understanding these and other human factors, a healthcare practitioner can truly learn and grow from within. The debriefing role is nonjudgemental and should guide the student through what they actually did, the thought processes they had and to reflect about whether they could have done anything differently.

DEBRIEF

According to Jaye et al. (2015), there are essentially three phases to a debrief: description, analysis and application. Initially, in the description phase, the facilitator will need to set the scene so everyone—the candidates, observers and tutor/facilitators—understands what happened in the simulation, ensuring that the same mental picture is shared or are all reading from the same hymn sheet. In addition, the facilitator needs to make it quite clear that the debrief session is a safe learning environment and that everyone respects each other and without judgement regarding the pass or fail criteria. The discussion is kept neutral and emotional responses avoided, especially for perceived poor performance.

MODEL DEBRIEFING QUESTIONS

'When you entered the scenario, what were your thoughts and feelings, and did you have an initial plan?'
   'The student nurse then told you the blood pressure was dropping so what was going through your mind and what happened?'
   'So, you gave fluid and started oxygen; then what happened?'
   'You were worried that the blood pressure was not improving and then what happened? And then what happened next?'

You should keep asking questions until you are confident that the details of the scenario have been fully highlighted for all the candidates and observers. If emotional responses are brought up, especially relating to poor performance, the facilitators need to stop this by making statements such as 'Let us not jump to any judgements right now about any perceived shortfalls, let us focus on what happened'.

The next stage is the analysis, where most of the learning happens. You need to spend most of the time in this phase, during which we deconstruct thoughts and actions of candidates and try to frame them around either nontechnical skills, wider human factors or clinical knowledge. Affective or emotional responses must be accepted and validated. As a result, if the student lost control of the situation or felt out of their depth, address this as an authentic emotion or thought, such as:

'We can all understand your predicament, I too during my clinical practice was put in a very similar position and felt the same way', or

'Your feelings are totally understandable, and most candidates feel the same way during this scenario'.

During analysis, we ask about the inner thoughts and feelings of the candidate; why they acted the way they did. Useful questions include:

'So, when the outreach team refused to come straight away, how did that make you feel? And why?'

'You tried to maintain the blood pressure until more helped arrived. How did you do that and why did you respond in the way you did?'

'It seemed like that you were having a real problem with the patient going into shock and help was not forth coming. Did it feel like that to you? What were your priorities during this time?'

'What I am hearing from you is during the scenario the blood pressure was not responding to the fluid challenges/boluses and you needed the outreach team but they were busy and could not come, is that right? How did that make you feel?'

'Did you consider other options?'

'Did you have another plan?'

'Could you have done anything else to guide or help you? Could you have asked anyone else for help and assistance?'

At this stage, use silence after questions to allow the candidates to think before they speak. Reflect key issues and responses back to the students to allow them to amend their responses. Keep the discussion polite and positive and avoid judgements on strengths and weaknesses. Try to allow the student to work out whether, upon reflection, they could have handled the scenario better. It is through this reflection that learning can be achieved and students can be more self-aware of how their internal environment can be affected by the external environment and vice-versa. By being more self-aware, healthcare practitioners can appreciate how and why they react and how their responses can improve when reacting to urgent or stressful situations in the future.

Facilitator: 'So my understanding is that outreach were delayed and the fluid was not supporting the blood pressure and the patient was going into peri-arrest; was that right?'

Candidate: 'Yes, I was really worried. After the second bag of 500 mLs of saline the blood pressure was still low, and I was desperate for the outreach team to come and help'.

Facilitator: 'So the patient was losing blood causing the blood pressure to drop. Could you have given anything else?'

At this point the facilitator should use silence to allow the candidate to reflect and think of possibilities.

Candidate: 'I could have given blood'!

Facilitator: 'Absolutely. The department has four units of O negative blood and in addition you can also activate the massive haemorrhage protocol'.

Candidate: 'Of course! I can't believe I missed that'!

Facilitator: 'Occasionally, in stressful situations, we cannot see the wider picture and we become less situationally aware—we become fixated. In this case, you just got fixated on the saline and you could not think of other options. This is really common, and we all do it. In situations like this when you are leading a team, it is always good to have a little huddle and quickly review the situation. In the scenario, you were not alone. You were the team leader, and in your team you had another nurse, a student nurse and a nursing assistant. Having a quick appraisal of what is happening can be really helpful because other team members will suggest options and take some of the stress away from you'.

Candidate: 'Yes, I definitely can see that now'.

Facilitator: 'So, to recap, we need to be more aware of how we make a plan of action, especially when things are not working as well as we hoped. We need time to think, reflect and communicate with the team about what is happening; and can we do anything else? In addition, we have guidelines and protocols for lots of medical emergencies that can help and give guidance'.

In the final stage, termed application, the facilitator focuses on how new learning can be applied to the wider clinical practice. Some helpful questions that you can ask are:

'What other situations can you think of that might be similar to the one in the scenario?'

'By understanding human factors little bit more now, how will this better your practice?'

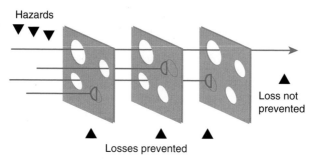

Fig. 5.1   Swiss cheese model of accident causation.

Finally, the facilitator should ask how what was learned from the scenario directly affects their practice tomorrow.

Facilitator: 'So how will the experience today affect your practice from now onwards?'

Candidate: 'Firstly, communicate with my team a lot more and periodically have a quick huddle to discuss the situation. In addition, if outreach cannot come immediately, consider other options such as calling the medical team and if the patient is in peri-arrest or deteriorating rapidly then I need to call the cardiac arrest team. Finally, consult trusted guidelines and protocols to assist me with charting a course of action and to determine current best practice'.

Before I conclude this chapter, I want to revisit the Bromiley case which I discussed in the beginning. In the Bromiley case, we saw a medical emergency of 'can't oxygenate can't intubate'. This unfortunate incident took place in 2005, and you could easily assume that this event occurred due to a unique set of circumstance that only pertained to that hospital, in that particular clinic, at that particular time. This tragic case could have been due to an unfortunate series of unique events that happened in a particular way or order for the incident to take place. In other words, the stars were aligned for this happen. This idea of a series of events that led to an undesirable incident has been described by James Reason as the Swiss cheese model of accident causation (Stein and Heiss, 2015) (Fig. 5.1).

If we examine other cases of medical errors worldwide, we will find causative influences that include human factors and nontechnical skills. Again, the practitioners involved would be senior, highly trained and proficient. Therefore, it is not a lack of clinical skills that leads to these medical emergencies but rather a lack of awareness of nontechnical skills such as communication, situational awareness and leadership. These cases, which are separated by time and geography, highlight that a lack of awareness of human factors and nontechnical skills can lead to unfavourable outcomes and increase medical complications over time and location. Only by accepting the role of human factors and placing a high importance on them in healthcare education can we begin to build safer clinical environments.

Conclusion

We have discussed the causal impacts to patient safety arising from nonappreciation of human factors and nontechnical skills. If clinicians do not learn and appreciate what human factors and nontechnical skills are and how they can potentially negatively impact clinical practice, then patient safety will be reduced and there will be an increase in risk and likelihood of errors. We have seen that we already have a wide range of assessment tools available to evaluate nontechnical skills, should we choose to use them. We have considered the challenges faced by education establishments in placing simulations in the curriculums to promote the learning of nontechnical skills. However, using technologies such as virtual reality and virtual patients can be a potential answer to overcome these difficulties. Any teaching programmes incorporating simulations require skilled and trained facilitators to ensure learning outcomes are met and to guide reflection so that students can internalise learning and become more self-aware. By incorporating simulations in healthcare training, practitioners can develop a deeper understanding of nontechnical skills and wider human factors. This understanding will better prepare practitioners to meet the increasing demands of modern healthcare, increase patient safety and cope with stressful situations.

Appendix 1

Simulation Example:

The candidate enters the simulation, is explained the brief and is asked to assess or treat the patient.

The candidate will have a staff team of three (any mix of RN, AN, physiotherapist, occupational therapist or HCA).

The candidate can ring any doctor (played by the simulation team) for any advice.

The candidate will need to assess and treat the patient using a systematic approach utilising the team effectively.

The simulation has three phases:

- Assessment
- Treatment
- Posttreatment scenarios A and B—depending on appropriateness of the treatment

Simulation	*Sepsis (either high or low fidelity)*
Phase 1	
Scenario brief	Mrs. Winston arrived in your department a few hours ago, via 999 ambulance, due to low blood pressure and reduced consciousness. Patient is drowsy, generally feeling unwell and has a chesty productive cough.
Social and medical history	Patient is 78 years old, lives in a nursing home. She had a right sided CVA 5 years ago, requires full care, is bed bound, has COPD (emphysema) diagnosed 10 years ago and a BMI of 35.6. Partner sadly died 15 years ago. She has one daughter who lives and works in Canada.
Assessment	
Safety aspects	Wash hands
	Students needs to wear AGP PPE until negative COVID-19 result
	Introduce themselves
	Check three points patient ID (ensure it is the correct patient)
A–E Assessment	
Airway	
	Clear. Patient has productive cough, drowsy but talking with no added sounds (e.g. no wheeze, no stridor). Can complete sentence in one breath.
Breathing	Saturations 90%, respiratory rate 22, chest expansion is equal. Auscultation: crackles are heard to lower and mid zones, normal resonance on percussion, trachea central. Not using accessory muscles.

Simulation	*Sepsis (either high or low fidelity)*
Circulation	Cap refill time 4 seconds, pulse is weak at radial site but at brachial site is 125 beats per minute. Blood pressure 95/58 mmHg, temperature 39.2°C. No neck vessel distension (no raised JVP), Heart sounds normal; ECG, if taken, shows sinus bradycardia. Urine output is reduced (if asked, the patient states that they have not been going as often as normal to empty bladder in the last 2 days).
Disability	Capillary blood glucose: 6.7. Patient is alert on ACVPU; 15/15 GCS. Pupils reacting equally to light and are not abnormal; no history of seizures.
Exposure	Patient is cool at peripheries but warm and a little clammy centrally. Otherwise, no rashes, swelling, deformity or masses to abdomen; bowel sounds present. No PR or PV bleeding. Patient has no IV drugs or fluids going through and no medications have been given yet.

Phase 2	After initial assessment
Candidate should consider:	Give reassurance to reduce anxiety.
The candidate will need to delegate some tasks to other members of the team such as the doctor, other nurses, including nursing associates and nursing assistants.	Increased anxiety could lead to elevated heart rate and respiratory rate.
Actions in bold are part of sepsis six protocol	Sit the patient up to help with breathing.
	COVID-19 PCR test
	Obtain sputum sample for microbiology
	Chest X-ray
	ECG
	Start oxygen
	Cannulation
	Take blood: U&Es, FBC, clotting screen
	Call and escalate to doctor using SBAR handover
	Commence fluids
	Place on hourly observations
	Work out NEWS score
	Blood culture
	Arterial blood gas (for respiratory function and **lactate**)
	Catheterise and **start strict fluid balance**
	Start broad spectrum antibiotic
	Call the outreach/deteriorating adult team
	Call ITU for support and advice
	Approximately 10% of patients with red flag sepsis will require ITU support

Blood and other results

All blood results are within acceptable except

Lactate	6
pO_2	9.5
pCO_2	8.0
pH	7.2
HCO_3	17
Chest X-ray	Shows pneumonia
ECG	Shows sinus tachycardia

Phase 3a

If treatment is given in a timely fashion, the patient does not deteriorate but remains critically unwell.

Treatment arm

The candidate will need to call the senior doctor and discuss that the patient is not improving.

Discussion should be about ceiling of treatment and a treatment plan, which should be continuation with sepsis six.

A referral to ITU could be sought, to see if ITU admission is a possibility if further deterioration occurs. If a referral is sought, the patient will not be a candidate for ITU admission due to past medical history.

The candidate needs to realise that the patient is critically unwell, not responding to treatment and is likely to deteriorate and a plan needs to be made accordingly.

Ceiling of treatment needs to be discussed, including respiratory and cardiac support. Intubation and inotropes are not possible as the patient is not eligible for ITU.

A key decision will revolve around DNAR/ReSPECT forms.

Contact the next of kin and inform them of the current situation.

Once the candidate speaks to the family member (breaking bad news), the scenario ends.

Debrief at end of simulation whether 3a or 3b.

Phase 3b

If treatment is not given in a timely fashion, the patient will deteriorate and arrest.

Nontreatment arm

The patient will arrest. The candidate will have to use the team to:

Phase 3b	*Nontreatment arm*
	Confirm cardiac arrest using an ABC approach
	Start chest compressions and summon help
	Ensure airway is maintained and the cardiac arrest team is called (ringing 2222)
	Defib pads are applied, and rhythm assessed
	1st rhythm PEA (give adrenaline)
	2nd rhythm asystole
	After the second asystole rhythm, the arrest team leader (played by facilitator) comes in to take a handover and then the simulation will finish.
	Debrief at end of simulation whether 3A or 3B

Human factors to consider	
Situational awareness	Has there been awareness of what is happening in the scenario, what is being done and what needs to be done? Is there awareness of changes in the evolving scenario and is there willingness to change the plan as more information is received?
Team working	Candidate asks team members their name, role and skill set. Team members are allocated tasks that are appropriate to their skill set. Performs regular huddles to keep team updated and asks for suggestions.
Decision-making	Prepared to make timely decisions regarding patient management. Has a plan if original plan is not succeeding and is willing to change any plan based on new information. Utilises trust, national guidelines and protocols for references to make sound decisions.
Priorities	Clearly spells out the priorities to the team regarding patient management. Priorities are based on logical and appropriate ranking. Candidate is willing to change the priorities based on new information.
Communication	Clearly communicates the plan to the team. Identifies which team members complete which tasks and asks confirmation when tasks are done. Reacts to results or new information and appropriately communicates this to the team. Has accurate verbal and written communications. Utilises communication aids, such as feedback loops when working with the team, SBAR when speaking to senior doctors and a communication tool such as SPIKES to break bad news.
Leadership	Clearly demonstrates to the team that they are leading the scenario and all information is channelled through them. All decisions are directed by them. Remains leader and does not get involved in tasks and keeps an overview and global perspective.
Problem-solving	The candidate users a systematic approach to assessing the patient's condition (A–E assessment). Utilises protocols and guidelines, such as sepsis six and ALS algorithm to initiate appropriate interventions.

References

Cooper, S., Cant, R., Porter, J., Sellick, K., Somers, G., Kinsman, L., et al., 2010. Rating medical emergency teamwork performance: development of the team emergency assessment measure (TEAM). Resuscitation 81 (4), 446–452.

Flin, R., O'Connor, P., Crichton, M., 2008. Safety at the Sharp End: A Guide to Non-technical Skills. Ashgate Publishing Company, Burlington.

Frenk, J., Chen, L., Bhutta, Z.A., Cohen, J., Crisp, N., Evans, T., et al., 2010. Health professionals for a new century: transforming education to strengthen health systems in an interdependent world. Lancet 376 (9756), 1923–1958.

Gjeraa, K., Jepsen, R.M., Rewers, M., Østergaard, D., Dieckmann, P., 2016. Exploring the relationship between anaesthesiologists' non-technical and technical skills. Acta Anaesthesiol. Scand. 60 (1), 36–47.

Glavin, R.J., Maran, N.J., 2003. Integrating human factors into the medical curriculum. Med. Educ. 37 (Suppl. 1), 59–64.

Higham, H., Greig, P.R., Rutherford, J., Vincent, L., Young, D., Vincent, C., 2019. Observer-based tools for non-technical skills assessment in simulated and real clinical environments in healthcare: a systematic review. BMJ Qual. Saf. 28 (8), 672–686.

Jaye, P., Thomas, L., Reedy, G., 2015. 'The Diamond': a structure for simulation debrief. Clin. Teach. 12 (3), 171–175.

Kim, J., Neilipovitz, D., Cardinal, P., Chiu, M., Clinch, J., 2006. A pilot study using high-fidelity simulation to formally evaluate performance in the resuscitation of critically ill patients: the University of Ottawa Critical Care Medicine, High-Fidelity Simulation, and Crisis Resource Management I Study. Crit. Care Med. 34 (38), 2167–2174.

Larsson, J., Holmström, I.K., 2013. How excellent anaesthetists perform in the operating theatre: a qualitative study on non-technical skills. Br. J. Anaesth. 110 (1), 115–121.

Lyk-Jensen, H.T., Jepsen, R.M., Spanager, L., Dieckmann, P., Ostergaard, D., 2014. Assessing nurse anaesthetists' non-technical skills in the operating room. Acta Anaesthesiol. Scand. 58 (7), 794–801.

Merry, A.F., 2007. Human factors and the cardiac surgical team: a role for simulation. J. Extra Corpor. Technol. 39 (4), 264–266.

Mitchell, L., Flin, R., Yule, S., Mitchell, J., Coutts, K., Youngson, G., 2012. Evaluation of the scrub practitioners' list of intraoperative non-technical skills system. Int. J. Nurs. Stud. 49 (2), 201–211.

Morgan, P.J., Tarshis, J., LeBlanc, V., Cleave-Hogg, D., DeSousa, S., Haley, M.F., et al., 2009. Efficacy of high-fidelity simulation debriefing on performance of practicing anaesthetist in simulated scenarios. Br. J. Anaesth. 103 (4), 531–537.

Peddle, M., 2015. Virtual simulation developing non-technical skills in student nurses and midwives. Aust. Nurs. Midwifery J. 23 (1), 41.

Peddle, M., Bearman, M., McKenna, L., Nestel, D., 2020. 'Getting it wrong to get it right': faculty perspectives of learning non-technical skills via virtual patient interactions. Nurse Educ. Today 88, 104381.

Pires, S., Monteiro, S., Pereira, A., Chaló, D., Melo, E., Rodrigues, A., 2017. Non-technical skills assessment for pre licensure nursing students: an integrative review. Nurse Educ. Today 58, 19–24.

Sevdalis, N., Davis, R., Koutantji, M., Undre, S., Darzi, A., Vincent, C.A., 2008. Reliability of a revised NOTECHS scale for use in surgical team. Am. J. Surg. 196 (2), 184–190.

Stein, J.E., Heiss, K., 2015. The Swiss cheese model of adverse event occurrence—closing the holes. Semin. Pediatr. Surg. 24 (6), 278–282.

Steinemann, S., Berg, B., DiTulio, A., Skinner, A., Terada, K., Anzelon, K., et al., 2012. Assessing teamwork in the trauma bay: introduction of a modified 'NOTECHS' scale for trauma. Am. J. Surg. 203 (1), 69–75.

Stiglich, J.M., 2019. Non-technical Skills Help Reduce Surgical Errors. Ocular Surgery News. https://www.healio.com/news/ophthalmology/20190315/nontechnical-skills-help-reduce-surgical-errors.

Wauben, L.S., Dekker-van Doorn, C.M., van Wijngaarden, J.D., Goossens, R.H., Huijsman, R., Klein, J., et al., 2011. Discrepant perceptions of communication, teamwork and situation awareness among surgical team members. Int. J. Qual. Health Care 23 (2), 159–166.

Westli, H.K., Johnsen, B.H., Eid, J., Rasten, I., Brattebø, G., 2010. Teamwork skills, shared mental models and performance in simulated trauma teams: an independent group design. Scand. J. Trauma Resusc. Emerg. Med. 18, 47.

White, N., 2012. Understanding the role of non-technical skills in patient safety. Nurs. Stand. 26 (26), 43–48.

Zausig, Y.A., Grube, C., Boeker-Blum, T., Busch, C.J., Bayer, Y., Sinner, B., et al., 2009. Inefficacy of simulator-based training on anaesthesiologists' non-technical skills. Acta Anaesthesiol. Scand. 53 (5), 611–619.

CHAPTER 6

Teamwork in Healthcare

Ally Ackbarally

CHAPTER AIMS

1. Meaning of team
2. Building a team
3. Team formation
4. Teamwork
5. Team communication
6. Team situation awareness
7. Team development

Introduction

Teamwork in healthcare is essential to maintain patient safety, ensure care quality and function well during critical or emergency situations in a very complex system. The need for people to work as a team is crucial in many industries, sports and in many walks of life to achieve a common goal or outcome, save lives and preserve safety. Teamwork is not only required in urgent or emergency situations but is also essential at all times because all patients in a hospital are unwell to different degrees and health outcomes depend heavily on teamwork. For example, if a surgeon and anaesthetist decide to operate on a patient who will likely need an intensive care bed without talking to the intensivist, they will put the patient in harm's way if there are no intensive care beds available postoperatively. Furthermore, teamwork is the one area in human factors wherein the whole team fails when other nontechnical skills such as communication, situation awareness or leadership fail. The Nursing and Midwifery Council (NMC, 2018) and the Health and Care Professions Council (HCPC, 2018) ensure that registrants work collaboratively as a team. To achieve this, you must:

- Respect the skills, expertise and contributions of your colleagues, referring matters to them when appropriate
- Maintain effective communication with colleague
- Keep colleagues informed when you are sharing the care of individuals with other health and care professionals and staff
- Work with colleagues to evaluate the quality of your work and that of the team
- Work with colleagues to preserve the safety of those receiving care
- Share information to identify and reduce risk
- Be supportive of colleagues who are encountering health or performance problems. However, this support must never compromise or be at the expense of patient or public safety (NMC, 2018, p. 11).

What Is a Team?

Teams are known to be a key feature component of organisations, high-risk industries, high demand team sports such as Formula One and football and, of course, healthcare. Teams are not usually uniform; they comprise groups of people with different skill sets, expertise, personalities, culture, resilience, and communication and leadership skills who are meant to work together to achieve the same goals, objectives and outcomes. Some are very good at it, owing to years of practice, coaching, team assessment or working together. In elite football, for example, coaches inculcate in their players a team mentality, teamwork, team ethic, situation awareness, communication, mutual support on the field, leadership skills of the players on an off the field, covering for each other and remaining a tight unit when under pressure. Conversely, in healthcare, very few teams undergo team training or team development regarding human factors, errors, nontechnical skills, safety improvement or being proactive to build the same mental model per Patient Safety II, especially teams at an operational level of 10–12 members or ward/departmental level. Some of the many reasons why teams do not always live up to the expectations are a lack of teamwork, inadequate communication, lack of leadership and confusing objectives such as a lack of role clarity during a crisis. Arguably, it is unrealistic to simultaneously train everyone who has been involved with a patient who needed below knee amputation (BKA) following a road traffic accident (RTA) which included the call operators, ambulance and paramedic crews, accident and emergency (A&E) teams, theatre teams, recovery teams, trauma wards, rehabilitation units, physiotherapy and community teams—to name a few. However, the National Confidential Enquiry into Patient Outcome and Death (NCEPOD, 2014) still recommends that professionals involved in patient care work together. As such, Salas et al. (1992, p. 4) define a team as a 'distinguishable set of two or more people who interact, dynamically, interdependent, and adaptively toward a common and valued goal/objective, mission, who have each been assigned specific roles or functions to perform, and who have limited life-span of membership'.

Working as a team has many benefits in healthcare systems. Table 6.1 presents examples of peer supervision, mutual support, productivity, efficiency and accountability (not to be confused with blame/punishment) of individual team members and of course to the patients because roles, tasks and responsibilities are well known. The Royal College of Physicians (2017, p. 3) acknowledges these by defining team as 'a small number of people with complementary skills who are committed to a common purpose, performance goals and approach for which they hold each other mutually accountable'.

Building a Team

In healthcare, we do not necessarily build a team, we mostly fill vacancies. Candidates need to possess the right skills, knowledge and experiences; but what about attitudes, work ethics, support and working and fitting into the team? It may be argued that it is difficult to assess or determine the emotional intelligence of candidates. However, this is something we must consider, especially in high-risk areas. Assessing emotional intelligence can also be considered a prerequisite in other clinical areas and administrative teams. Two examples of core teams in clinical environments are shown in Figs 6.1 and 6.2.

TABLE 6.1 ■ Advantages of Effective/Good Teams in Healthcare Examples

Patient	Organisational Level	Local Level
• Improved patient safety • Reduced errors • Reduced incidents • Improvement in quality of care • Improved communication with patient • Patient at the centre of care and safety • Safety culture • Less mortality and morbidity • Improved patient satisfaction	• Good teamwork usually means organisational success (Rosen et al., 2018) • Clinical effectiveness • Cost effectiveness • Better committed staff • Better staff retention • Cost savings • Safety culture • Easier for change to take place • Easier to align organisational strategies, values and visions	• Mutual support • Peer support • Peer review • Improved efficiency • Improved effectiveness • Continuity • Skilled workforce • Reduce stress • Reduce ill health • Happier workforce (cannot be underestimated) • Mutual trust • Mutual respect • Safety culture • Formation of local norms and values based on mutual respect • Reduce and solve conflicts • Better coordination • Easier to speak up • Easier to question • Easier to lead • Generating ideas • Responsive • Improved performances both individually and as teams

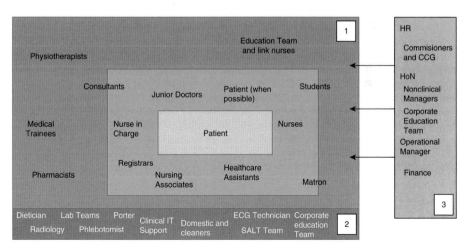

Fig. 6.1　Core clinical team. *CCG,* Clinical commissioning group; *ECG,* electrocardiographic; *IT,* information technology; *SALT,* *S*ort, assess, *L*ifesaving interventions, *T*reatment and/or transport.

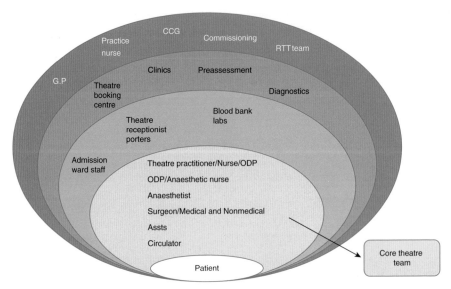

Fig. 6.2 Operating theatre team. ODP, Operating department practitioner.

In Fig. 6.1, Team 1 represents a core clinical team; this team comprises people closest to the patients. They are usually a consistent team and will know the patients best. Team 2 is also essential for patient care and support and is crucial in supporting the core team. Team 3 can also influence patient care and their decisions will affect clinical output and safety. For example, if the operational manager and head of nursing (HoN) decided to make general savings before the end of the financial and agreed with human resources (HR) and finance to withhold recruiting funds, the staff workload would increase and they would feel pressured and stressed—inadvertently leading to unsafe practice and errors as discussed in other chapters. Staff usually perceive these events as an outside influence.

Furthermore, the core team (which should also include patients when possible) consists of individuals who have constant input in patient care and consequently will have a greater influence on quality and safety. Team 2 members such as porters, domestic workers or lab personnel will interact with the core team regarding communications, patient transfers or blood results, among other tasks; other members such as the physiologists and pharmacists may interact directly with the patients.

Other individuals will influence the core team regarding patient safety, such as how the matron leads the unit and influences the team culture. Other departments, including finance, can also influence the core team concerning resources or staff well-being. These are only a few examples.

Fig. 6.2 illustrates teams and teamwork that are interdependent when it comes to all aspects of patient safety. For example, the core team has to work closely with each other in the physical sense and as a unit because all members need to be present most of the time. In addition, they need to establish mental closeness, meaning sharing the same mental model (discussed further in the chapter), so that the entire theatre team is working towards the same goals, especially in critical moments or emergency situations. Due to the high-risk elements of surgery and anaesthesia, these departments have adopted tools such as a theatre safety checklist to enable development of the right working culture, especially concerning safety, quality and communications. Despite these measures, the theatre team can still make a mistake which is why nontechnical elements and teamwork are important in moments when patients are at the most risk. However, unlike ward areas where the patients are in one place, the surgical journey can be hazardous for

EXERCISE 6.1

> HCPC (2018)
> Work with colleagues
> 2.5 You must work in partnership with colleagues, sharing your skills, knowledge and experience where appropriate, for the benefit of service users and carers.
>
> 2.6 You must share relevant information, where appropriate, with colleagues involved in the care, treatment or other services provided to a service user.

In healthcare, wherever you work and whatever your job and roles are, you will work as part of a team. You may work with a consistent team or in places where there are different teams regularly. You may think you work in a great team or a team that needs improvement. It is always helpful to critically reflect on your team by looking at the positive aspects and those that need improvement.

Step 1
Questions you may want to ask yourself about your team.

1.
If you are not happy with your team and do not feel supported, you may want to consider asking specific questions to see if your team shows any signs of dysfunctions as demonstrated below (Fig. 6.3):

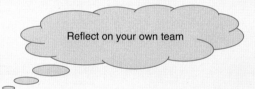

Reflect on your own team

2.
The assessment checklist may provide a different perspective and an objective view of the team. The following checklist, adapted from Health Education England (n.d.) will help you conduct an assessment of your team (Royal College of Physicians, 2017).

1. Are team members clear about what we are trying to achieve?
2. Can we rely on one another? Do we work supportively to get the job done?
3. Do we have lively debates about how best to work?
4. Do we meet sufficiently often to ensure effective communication and cooperation?
5. Are people in the team quick to offer help and find new ways of doing things?
6. Do we all have influence on final decisions?
7. Are we careful to keep each other informed about work issues?
8. Is there a feeling of trust and safety in this team?
9. Are we enthusiastic about innovation?
10. Are team members committed to achieving the set objectives?
11. Can we safely discuss errors and mistakes?
12. Is there is a climate of constructive criticism in this team?

Step 2

Now that you have a better understanding of your team, including its strengths and weaknesses, you may want to consider the following to help you build a better team:

1. Highlight the positives of the team to the members.
2. What development does your team need?
3. Will team building exercises help?
4. How do you address the weaknesses?
5. Has the team acknowledged their weaknesses?
6. Who can help?
7. When to start with what?
8. What are the barriers?
9. Are the opportunities defined, clear and acknowledged?
10. Can we agree on the team vision, goals and objectives?
11. Focus on issues and not individuals.
12. What is the one thing the team needs to stop doing and the one thing the team needs to start doing?

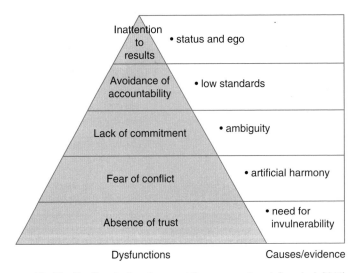

Fig. 6.3   The five dysfunctions and the causes of each (Lencioni, 2011).

patients travelling through different departments in the community to hospitals and theatre departments. If initial pathway errors occur, they may corkscrew down to the day of surgery. The theatre team is very reliant on the other teams to get everything right. Inter-teamwork and strong communication channels (verbal and written) are very important for team situational awareness.

The resuscitation team (Fig. 6.4) is quite different from the theatre team whose members are relatively familiar with each other and the ward core team, in most cases. Usually, a resuscitation team comprises a group of people with the training and skills to visit different areas of a hospital

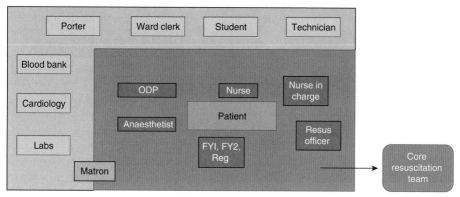

Fig. 6.4 Resuscitation in clinical areas. *FY1, 2, Foundation year 1, 2 (doctors).*

to support or lead a cardiac arrest or other emergencies. The team will include resuscitation officers who are unfamiliar with the clinical areas, an anaesthetist and an operating department practitioner (ODP) who do not work with each other often or are new staff members on the ward who are not fully confident with their surroundings and the prevailing system. Indeed, resuscitation skills are crucial in a cardiac arrest situation; however, the importance of nontechnical skills, which are the elements that affects our performances in all situations, are now acknowledged as crucial in emergency medicine. For example, the anaesthetist does not know the patient, and the speciality doctors do not know the anaesthetist or nurses very well; nevertheless, they have to work together (probably) for the first time in an emergency situation to save a patient. This is when team leadership, communication and situational awareness are vital to maintain team cohesion, and where collaboration and cooperation will enhance teamwork. Any poor performances of these nontechnical skills by a team or an individual will have an effect on patient outcomes.

Team Formation

A team needs to be nurtured, supported, coached and developed so that it becomes supportive, shares the same mental model and is resilient to errors and mistakes. This can be achieved over time by a supportive leader with a clear vision and strategy that all members believe in. The process of team building or team forming proposed by Tuckman (1965) and Tuckman and Jensen (1977) are still widely accepted today (Fig. 6.5).

Especially in healthcare, not all teams will need to move through all first four stages of development. For example, a theatre operating team or a paramedic crew may not have to go through the storming stage because there are already guidelines, policies and procedures that the team needs to follow. In healthcare, the stages of team building are complex and may not follow the stages that Tuckman (1965) envisaged—although it is a good visual template to situate the team.

However, in emergency situations where arrivals of individuals are staggered, team members may not have met before and individual skills are not always fully known, it is crucial to promote teamwork. The responding team will not have the luxury to go through the team processes but will have to quickly gather information for team situation awareness and

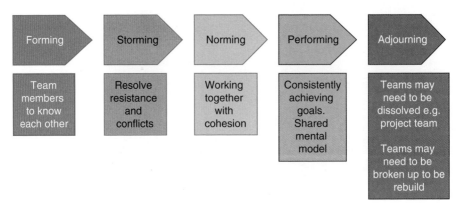

Fig. 6.5 Team formation and dissolution stages.

decision-making, decide on leadership, establish communication and tasks and work as a team under stressful situations. This is no mean feat under normal situations, let alone in emergency situations.

To achieve team efficiency and performance in those circumstances, more than tasks and teamwork need to be achieved. Taskwork and teamwork behaviours are both essentials and have to be correct and properly executed. Taskwork behaviours are more than technical tasks; they include understanding the need for the tasks or the operating procedures (Salas et al., 2007, 2008). Salas et al. (2007, 2008) argue that teamwork behaviours are about how the individual team members make sure that the team is performing and functioning as a cohesive unit including cooperating and coordinating effectively, mutually supporting and providing feedback to each other. This is when a team becomes efficient and safe. Moreover, Salas et al. (2000) claim that specific team behaviours and norms are critical for optimum team performance (Table 6.2).

Teamwork

It is a well-established fact that teamwork is a prognosticator of success and positive outcomes in sports, high risk industries, aviation and healthcare. Many analyses and research confirm this in the literature. In healthcare, teamwork is crucial because the system is very complex; it normally involves several departmental layers separated not only by walls but also in the way people work, communicate and deliver care. There are normally many people—clinicians and nonclinicians—involved in patient care; this can potentially increase risks to patients regarding error probability and miscommunications. Effective teamwork in healthcare has a direct effect on patient outcomes,

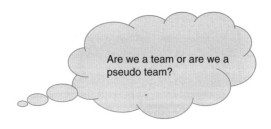

TABLE 6.2 ■ Teamwork Behaviours and Performance Norms

	Dimensions	Definitions
Teamwork behaviour	Performance monitoring	Team members observe the behaviour of their team members and accept that their own behaviour is being observed or monitored
	Feedback	A climate in which feedback is offered and accepted among members
	Closed-loop communication	Message is sent, feedback provided and verified for accuracy
	Backing-up behaviours	Team members have the competency and willingness to help and accept help from others
Team performance norms	Team self-awareness	The team members share the same values and feelings as their team members
	Fostering of team interdependence	Understanding that success depends on each other

Adapted from Salas et al. 2007, 2008.

as demonstrated by Weaver et al. (2014) and Zajac et al. (2021). More importantly, ineffective teamwork or lack of high-quality teamwork will lead to harm (Rowland, 2014) and adverse events, especially with pseudo-teams (West and Lyubovnikova, 2012). Sometimes, it is easy to believe that because we are working closely with other departments, professionals and people in the same unit, we are part of the same team. The reality can be very different; mental models, supervisors, leadership accountability, objectives and priorities can vary. This is when patients are at risk and errors can easily happen when the team does not meet the teamwork criteria of being supportive, communicating, coordinating and demonstrating good leadership.

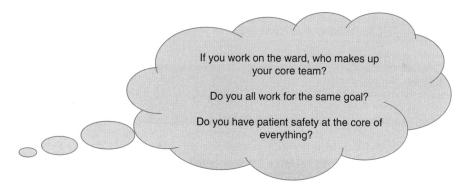

If you work on the ward, who makes up your core team?

Do you all work for the same goal?

Do you have patient safety at the core of everything?

Teamwork in healthcare is usually defined and described in rather broad terms such as work that requires the coordination and articulation of tasks and activities between a group of people (Salas et al., 2005). Rutherford et al. (2012) state the prerequisites of teamwork are supporting others, solving conflicts, exchanging information and coordinating activities. The Chartered Institute of Personnel and Development (CIPD) argues that teamwork is best achieved when the team shares the same goal, has a sense of purpose and exhibits these specific characteristics (Royal College of Physicians, 2017):

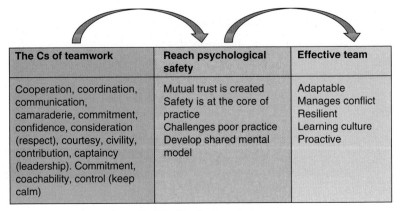

The Cs of teamwork	Reach psychological safety	Effective team
Cooperation, coordination, communication, camaraderie, commitment, confidence, consideration (respect), courtesy, civility, contribution, captaincy (leadership). Commitment, coachability, control (keep calm)	Mutual trust is created Safety is at the core of practice Challenges poor practice Develop shared mental model	Adaptable Manages conflict Resilient Learning culture Proactive

Fig. 6.6   Developing a team.

- Common sense of purpose
- Clear understanding of objectives
- Resources to achieve objectives
- Mutual respect among team members
- Value members' strengths and weaknesses
- Mutual trust
- Willingness to speak openly
- Range of skills to deal effectively with tasks
- Range of personal styles for team roles

These are the elements and characteristics that need careful consideration when assessing team performance and building a team (Fig. 6.6).

CASE STUDY 6.1   An Example of Teamwork in Healthcare

A patient was admitted to theatre recovery following a post carotid endarterectomy. The patient had spent 3 hours in theatre recovery and was about to be discharged. The patient met all the discharge criteria and was physiologically stable, fully awake and alert. While handing over to the nurse, a trickle of arterial blood suddenly came through the Tegarderm dressing and light pressure was applied at the bleeding point. The recovery nurse asked another colleague to get another dressing and gauze to apply a pressure dressing. However, within seconds more blood was coming out and more pressure was applied. As the patient saw the blood, he panicked, blood pressure went up and suddenly it was a massive bleed. The emergency buzzer was pulled and the patient oxygen saturation dropped as he could not breathe. By this time, it was a scary scene, the recovery nurse was covered in blood and the patient's face and pillow were also covered in blood.

Two consultant anaesthetists arrived at the same time and no one took charge, coordinated or led. They both 'froze' (happens when cognitively overloaded). A third consultant anaesthetist arrived on the scene, assessed the situation and realised the team was 'stuck'. He calmly assumed the team lead role by reassuring everyone and then coordinated the tasks. One anaesthetist was instructed to sedate the patient while the other intubated the patient. Blood was started and the patient was rushed to the vascular theatre.

Reflection

What made the difference? Was it the team leader or collaboration?

Leadership and communication are the cornerstones of teamwork.

CASE STUDY 6.2	Lack of Teamwork in Eastern Airline Flight 401 on 29 December 1972

The Eastern Airlines Flight 401 was flying from New York to Miami, a regular route for the crew. The airplane for the flight was a new Lockheed L-1011-1 TriStar, which had been delivered to the airline on 18 August, 1972. The cockpit team comprised very experienced pilots with different experiences flying a Lockheed L-1011-1 TriStar.

'The flight was under the command of Captain Robert Albin (Bob) Loft, aged 55 years, a veteran pilot ranked 50th in seniority at Eastern Airlines. Captain Loft had been with the airline for 32 years and had accumulated a total of 29,700 flight hours throughout his flying career. He had logged 280 hours in the L-1011-1. His flight crew included First Officer Albert John (Bert) Stockstill, aged 39 years, who had 5800 hours of flying experience (with 306 of them in the L-1011-1), and Flight Engineer Donald Louis (Don) Repo, aged 51 years, who had 15,700 hours of flying experience, with 53 of them in the L-1011-1'.

The flight was 'routine' (you have heard this before, 'routine surgery') until the approach to Miami International Airport. The crew realised that the main landing gear lights were on but the nose wheel had not illuminated. The crew (whole team) got fixated onto this and eventually lost situation awareness, had no clear leadership in the cockpit and coordination and communication were poor. The plane lost almost 2000 feet of altitude in a few minutes without the crew/team noticing until it was too late.

The following conversation was recovered from the flight voice recorder:

Stockstill: 'We did something to the altitude'.

Loft: 'What'?

Stockstill: 'We're still at 2000 feet, right'?

Loft: 'Hey—what's happening here'?

Less than 10 seconds after this exchange, the plane crashed. Unfortunately, 104 out of 176 people died.

The National Transportation Safety Board (NTSB) in 1973 attributed the crash to 'the failure of the flight crew to monitor the flight instruments during the final 4 minutes of flight, and to detect an unexpected descent soon enough to prevent impact with the ground. Preoccupation with a malfunction of the nose landing gear position indicating system distracted the crew's attention from the instruments and allowed the descent to go unnoticed'.

In response to this incident, many airlines around the world started crew resource management training (team training) for their pilots. The training is designed to make problem solving in the cockpit much more efficient—thus causing less distraction for the crew.

National Transportation Safety Board, 1973. Aircraft Accident Report Eastern Airlines, Inc. Report Number: NTSB-AAR-73-14. https://www.ntsb.gov/investigations/AccidentReports/Reports/AAR7314.pdf (Accessed 30 October 2023).

Reflection

- Can you draw an analogy between this incident and the Bromiley case (Chapter 5, Nontechnical Skills)?
- Do you have team training in your department? Do you train together with a multidisciplinary team?
- Can you perceive how nontechnical skills are interrelated?

Team Communication

In the current highly complex healthcare systems, where a short stay for a minor procedure in the hospital may involve more than 20 people directly and indirectly in the delivery of care, communication in all its aspects (Chapter 7, Communication in Relation to Patient Safety) is the common thread to safety and effective teamwork. Patients will be handed over (handoffs) several times during the day to different multidisciplinary teams and departments. Team communication and collaboration are essential, and when communication is not effective, critical information for patient safety may be lost or changed by accidents which will put patients at risk. These could happen because of assumptions, misinterpretations, unclear communications or miscommunications. Effective team communication is not limited to patient safety; it has been associated with reduced stress, improved job satisfaction, staff retention and improved team and workplace trust (Weaver et al., 2014).

Communication barriers can be different for each team including hierarchy culture, interprofessional communications, unreliable technology, stress and fatigue. These can affect communications and the way a team communicates. Team members and team leaders must identify the barriers to their team communication and find their own creative solutions. Tools such as the situation, background, assessment and recommendation (SBAR) and collaborative ways of working using team briefs or huddles are easy yet effective solutions for improving team communication, as proven during coronavirus disease 2019 pandemic. Communication has to be right as it is the reason for most adverse or near miss incidents in acute settings. Poor quality communication will heighten team anxieties and stress levels which will reduce the team performance. Team training and team development using structured tools, huddles or briefing effectively will improve teamwork, performances and interprofessional communication as well as reduce hierarchical gradients. Careful consideration must be taken to ensure that team briefing, debriefing and huddles take place in areas where the team will not be disturbed or distracted so that members can completely focus on the information being discussed. The team briefings should be structured but also flexible and open enough to allow members to ask questions or clarify misunderstandings. TeamSTEPSS (Team Strategies and Tools to enhance performance and Patient Safety) (Agency for Healthcare Research and Quality, n.d.) recommends some key questions:

- Who is on the team?
- Does the team understand and agree about goals?
- Are roles and responsibilities understood?
- What is the plan of action/care?
- What is the staff availability during the shift? Who has responsibilities for other areas (e.g. the bleep holder for the department)?
- How will workload be shared among the staff we have?
- What resources are available during the shift?
- What issues/problems do we have today?

Communication also requires the safe handling of information and if this fails, it will have repercussions on the care and safety of patients. Healthcare providers, managers, team leaders and the education team need to ensure that communication training and team communication training are prioritised as communication is the common thread to safety. Team training, especially with a multidisciplinary team, will not only improve safe communication within the team but will also help overcome barriers, reduce hierarchy and facilitate psychological safety so that members will feel confident to question, challenge and endorse safe practice. Individually, the following steps can be considered to ensure safe and effective communication (Royal College of Physicians, 2017):

- Introduce yourself and clarify your role
- Listen attentively and allow people to complete their thoughts
- Ask questions for clarification
- Check for understanding of what has been said
- Invite opinions from those who have not spoken
- Be aware of communication barriers (e.g. hierarchy)
- Use objective not subjective language

- Show mutual respect
- Consider the setting (right place, adequate time, no distractions)
- Be aware of body language, both given and received (e.g. facial expressions, eye contact, posture)

Team Situation Awareness

Situation awareness (SA) is a nontechnical skill important to safety at both individual and team levels (Chapter 5, Nontechnical Skills). Simply put, SA is about being cognisant and knowing what is happening around you—physically, mentally and with regards to space and time—in this context during a team meeting. We do this all the time, sometimes without even realising it, such as when driving or walking. Ives and Hillier (2015, p. 6) define SA as 'the ability to identify, process and comprehend the critical elements of information in a dynamic situation, and be able to predict what will happen next'. In other words, do you know what happened, what is happening and what will likely happen next?

The same is true for team situation awareness (TSA). For example, is the team aware of what is happening, what instructions mean and how to identify stress? Have they noticed somebody struggling with a task or fixated on a specific task to the detriment of others? TSA, sometimes also referred to as 'shared SA', is defined as the point where all the team members have the same situational awareness of shared SA requirements (Endsley and Jones, 2001). The common SA requirements are what keep the team safe and working as one, especially in emergency situations. Wellens (1993) and Salas et al. (1995) hold similar views; TSA is believed to be the sharing of a common understanding between the team regarding current environmental events, their meaning and what can/will happen, underpinned by teamwork behaviours and cognitive processes which will enhance teamwork and team performances. Schulz et al. (2013) and She and Li (2017) also pointed out that team SA encompasses and requires the contribution of each individual member's SA. Although the team is a group of people with different skills and responsibilities, TSA is crucial for effective teamwork.

For example, if the surgeon asks for a Poole suction towards the end of surgery:

- Does everyone interpret this as a potential massive haemorrhage?
- Does everyone recognise the danger?
- Does everyone think of the massive haemorrhage protocol and act accordingly?
- Is communication about the situation clear within the team and does everybody know what to do?

If so, do they share the same mental model or mental image? Besides effective communication, TSA can be enhanced by new technologies such as a shared technology display wherein the whole team can see information such as the National Early Warning Score (NEWS) or blood results. These skills and abilities to process information and data and analyse what has happened, what is happening and what will happen come with training and working in a stable team underpinned by a strong workplace culture (see Chapter 10, Culture in the Workplace).

Team Development

No matter how effective the team is, continuous improvement and development is needed for the group and the individual members. Team development should consist of team training, team assessment and opportunities to deliberate, debrief, reassess goals and objectives and teamwork and team effectiveness discussions. However, these do not happen too often in healthcare; moreover, with the ongoing difficulties of the National Health Service (NHS) post pandemic and the chronic lack of staff, team training are not happening regularly. In the absence of regular team training such as problem solving by the team, simulation of a scenario or team activities, teams could consider Balint groups and Schwarz rounds as methods to facilitate reflections and improve cohesions. The (Royal College of Physicians, 2017) advises using a checklist to help teams discuss their development (Box 6.1).

BOX 6.1 ■ Checklist for Team Development

Objectives

- What are our current objectives/goals and why?
- Are they SMART (specific, measurable, attainable, relevant, time-bound)?
- Do they need to be updated or reviewed?
- What are we doing as a team to achieve our objectives?
- What does success look like?

Roles and responsibilities

Are all members aware of each other's roles and responsibilities moving forward?

Review and reflect/team innovation

- What have we done well?
- What could we have done better?
- What should we stop doing?
- What should we start doing?
- How can we work better together?

Rewarding individuals and teams

Are there any individuals or overall successes that team members would like to highlight?

Facilitated discussion on sharing stressful situations

Have there been difficult cases or problems that the team would like to discuss here or separately?

Identifying learning needs

- Have there been any changes to working practice or relevant guidelines/policy that the team should be aware of?
- Does the team have any learning needs that need to be addressed?

> Consider doing the checklist exercise and see what development the team needs?

Simulation is an effective way to develop, assess and evaluate the whole team (Rovamo et al, 2015). How many times do people say they are part of a great team or they feel the team is poor? How do we know what the truth is? Is there empirical evidence for what practitioners say? Most teams in healthcare are not 'assessed' empirically. Although there are no specific universal tools available, there are validated tools that can be used for specific teams. For example, theatre teams can be assessed using the Observational Teamwork Assessment for Surgery (OTAS), emergency teams may use the Team Emergency Assessment Measure (TEAM) (Cooper et al, 2016), teamwork in the clinical environment can be assessed using the Team Performance Observation Tool (TPOT) (Zhang et al., 2015) and obstetrics and gynaecology teams can use the Assessment of Obstetrical Team Performance (AOTP) (Morgan et al., 2012). However, tools are only one aspect of training and assessment; they need to be used judiciously and effectively so that they do not cause further confusion and issues.

Conclusion

Teams and individual team members are the cornerstones of patient care and safety; therefore, they must be nurtured, supported and improved upon to continuously provide the safest care. Leadership plays an important role in teams and teamwork; however, everyone in a team is a leader within their scope of practice and responsibilities. All members of a team must contribute and communicate effectively to heighten team SA, which enables the team to be safe and effective.

Key Points

- Teams can be developed
- Teams can be improved
- Teams can be assessed

References

Agency for Healthcare Research and Quality (AHRQ), n.d. https://www.ahrq.gov/research/publications/pubcomguide/index.html.

Cooper, et al., 2010. Rating medical emergency teamwork performance: Development of the Team Emergency Assessment Measure (TEAM). Simulation and Education 81 (40), 446–452. https://doi.org/10.1016/j.resuscitation.2009.11.027.

Endsley, M.R., Jones, W.M., 2001. A model of inter and intra team situational awareness: implications for design, training and measurement. New trends in cooperative activities: understanding system dynamics in complex environments. In: McNeese, M., Salsa, E., Endsley, M. (Eds.), New Trends in Cooperative Activities: Understanding System Dynamics in Complex Environments. Human Factors and Ergonomics Society, Santa Monica, pp. 46–68.

Health and Care Professionals Council (HCPC), 2018. Standards of Conduct, Performance and Ethics. https://www.hcpc-uk.org/standards/standards-of-conduct-performance-and-ethics/.

Health Education England, n.d. https://heeoe.hee.nhs.uk/sites/default/files/buildingtheteamchecklist_1.docx.

Ives, C., Hillier, S., 2015. Human Factors in Healthcare: Common Terms. 2015 Clinical Human Factors Group. www.chfg.org.

Lencioni, P., 2011. Five Dysfunctions of a Team. A Leadership Fable. http://5dysfunctions.blogspot.com/p/philosophy-assessment.html.

Morgan, P.J., Tregunno, D., Pittini, R., Tarshis, J., Regehr, G., Desousa, S., et al., 2012. Determination of the psychometric properties of a behavioural marking system for obstetrical team training using high-fidelity simulation. BMJ Qual. Saf. 21 (1), 78–82.

National Confidential Enquiry into Patient Outcome and Death (NCEPOD), 2014. Lower Limb Amputation: Working Together. https://www.ncepod.org.uk/2014lla.html.

National Transport Safety Board, 1973. File No. 1-0016. Aircraft Accident Report, Eastern Airlines Inc, L-1011, N310EA, Maimi Florida Dec 29, 1972. https://www.ntsb.gov/investigations/AccidentReports/Reports/AAR7314.pdf.

Nursing & Midwifery Council (NMC), 2018. The Code: Professional standards of practice and behaviour for nurses, midwives and nursing associates. http://www.nmc.org.uk/globalassets/sitedocuments/nmc-publications/revised-new-nmc-code.pdf.

Rosen, M.A., DiazGranados, D., Dietz, A.S., Benishek, L.E., Thompson, D., Pronovost, P.J., et al., 2018. Teamwork in healthcare: Key discoveries enabling safer, high-quality care. Am. Psychol 73 (4), 433–450.

Rovamo, L., Nurmi, E., Mattila, N.M., et al., 2015. Effect of a simulation-based workshop on multidisplinary teamwork of newborn emergencies: an intervention study. BMC Res Notes 8, 671. https://doi.org/10.1186/s13104-015-1654-2.

Rowland, P., 2014. Core principles and values of effective team-based health care. J. Interprof. Care 28 (1), 79–80.

Royal College of Physicians (RCP), 2017. Improving teams in healthcare. Resource 4: Team Development. Faculty of Medical Leadership and Management. NHS Health Education England.

Rutherford, J.S., Flin, R., Mitchell, L., 2012. Teamwork, communication, and anaesthetic assistance in Scotland. Brit. J. Anaesth. 109 (1), 21–26.

Salas, E., Cooke, N.J., Rosen, M.A., 2008. On Teams,Teamwork, and Team Performance: discoveries and Developments. Hum. Factors 50 (3), 540–547. https://doi.org/10.1518/001872008X288457.

Salas, E., Dickinson, T.L., Converse, S.A., Tannenbaum, S.I., 1992. Toward and understanding of team performance and training. In: Swezey, R.W., Salas, E. (Eds.), Teams: Their Training and Performance. Ablex, Norwood, pp. 3–29.

Salas, E., Prince, C., Baker, D.P., Shrestha, L., 1995. Situation awareness in team performance: implications for measurement and training. Hum. Factors 37 (1), 123–136.

Salas, E., Rhodenizer, L., Bowers, C.A., 2000. The design and delivery of crew resource management training: exploiting available resources. Hum. Factors 42 (3), 490–511.

Salas, E., Sims, D., Burke, C.S., 2005. Is There a 'Big Five' in Teamwork? Small Group Research 36 (5), 555–599. https://doi.org/10.1177/1046496405277134.

Salas, E., Stagl, K.C., Burke, C.S., Goodwin, G.F., 2007. Fostering Team Effectiveness in Organizations: Toward an Integrative Theoretical Framework of Team Performance. Nebraska Symposium on Motivation.

Schulz, C.M., Endsley, M.R., Kochs, E.F., Gelb, A.W., Wagner, K.J., 2013. Situation awareness in anaesthesia: concept and research. Anaesthesiology 18 (3), 729–742.

She, M., Li, Z., 2017. Team situation awareness: a review of definitions and conceptual models. In: Harris, D. (Ed.), Engineering Psychology and Cognitive Ergonomics: Performance, Emotion and Situation Awareness. EPCE 2017. Lecture Notes in Computer Science, vol. 10275. Springer, Cham.

Tuckman, B.W., 1965. Development sequence in small groups. Psychol. Bull. 63 (6), 384–399.

Tuckman, B.W., Jensen, M.A.C., 1977. Stages of small-group development revisited. Group Organ. Stud. 2 (4), 419–427.

Weaver, S.J., Dy, S.M., Rosen, M.A., 2014. Team-training in healthcare: a narrative synthesis of the literature. BMJ Qual. Saf. 23 (5), 359–372.

Wellens, A.R., 1993. Group situation awareness and distributed decision making: from military to civilian applications. In: Castellan, N.J. (Ed.), Individual and Group Decision Making. Psychology Press, London, pp. 267–291.

West, M.A., Lyubovnikova, J., 2012. Real teams or pseudo teams? The changing landscape needs a better map. Ind. Organ. Psychol. 5 (1), 25–55.

Zajac, S., Woods, A., Tannenbaum, S., Salas, E., Holladay, C.L., 2021. Overcoming challenges to teamwork in healthcare: a team effectiveness framework and evidence-based guidance. Front. Commun. 6, 1–20.

Zhang, C., Miller, C., Volkman, K., Meza, J., Jones, K., 2015. Evaluation of the team performance observation tool with targeted behavioral markers in simulation-based 32 interprofessional education. J. Interprof. Care 29 (3), 202–208.

CHAPTER 7

Communication in Relation to Patient Safety

Ally Ackbarally ▪ Kay De Vries

CHAPTER AIMS

1. Define communication skills and discuss their importance
2. Describe and discuss strategies to improve communication
3. Describe and discuss barriers to communication

Introduction

This chapter is presented in two sections. The first section discusses communication in practice with a focus on patient safety and its contextual application as a nontechnical skill that can reduce errors.

In the second section, advanced communication, importance of quality engagement and the relationship between healthcare professionals and patients when undertaking a psychosocial assessment are considered. This section draws on communication skill development within palliative care and oncology.

Communication is one of the most important components to ensure safe and quality care and plays a major role in effective and efficient teams. However, if communication fails, it will certainly lead to errors or potentially to major patient incidences.

Miscommunication, misinterpretation of communication, lack of or noncommunication, misreading verbal or nonverbal cues and confirmation bias are but a few examples of the main causes of incidences in healthcare settings. Furthermore, poor communication is among the top three complaints reported to the Parliamentary and Health Service Ombudsman (2019–20).

Tools are available to help mitigate communication issues; however, despite all best efforts, communication is still amongst the leading cause of errors in healthcare. Thus, there is much scope for improvement.

Section One

WHAT IS COMMUNICATION?

Ives and Hillier (2015) define communication as the process of passing information or instructions between people so that it is received and understood as intended (Box 7.1). Although this can be perceived as a simple definition, communication in healthcare is generally rather complex. It can also include the exchange of feelings in certain contexts, such as when challenging somebody, and establish predictable behaviour patterns (Flin et al., 2008). Communication is also vital for leadership, team dynamics, situation awareness and task management.

BOX 7.1 ▪ Piper Alpha Disaster

Late in the evening on 6 July, 1988, a series of explosions ripped through the Piper Alpha platform in the North Sea. Engulfed in fire, over the next few hours most of the oil rig topside modules collapsed into the sea; 167 men died. Although the enquiry blamed the disaster on poor facility maintenance, a closer look at the contributing factors revealed a catastrophic communication failure at the shift handover regarding informing the next shift that a pressure safety valve has been removed, which presumably led to the disaster from the actions taken by the night shift staff. In addition, failure to initially communicate with two other platforms feeding into the Piper Alpha after the explosions intensified the fire and made escapes and rescue much more difficult.

Failure to Communicate Blood Results

Just after 6:00 p.m. the ward clerk answered a phone call from a lab technician asking to speak with the nurse looking after Patient A. The ward clerk could not find Nurse T and wrote a message on a note pad regarding a high vancomycin level for Patient A. Just before the ward clerk was leaving the shift at 6:30 p.m., she found Nurse T and gave her the note and said it was about the drug levels for Patient A. As Nurse T was in the middle of a task and had gloves on, she put the note in her pocket with the intention to look at the note later. It was a busy late shift and the ward was short of a staff nurse, so it was busier than usual. Nurse T realised that the night shift staff were already in the unit waiting for handover at 7:00 p.m. She took her handover document and went to the office to handover her patients to the night shift staff, signed her documents and went home. At 8:45 p.m., Nurse T rang the ward and explained that she just found a note in her pocket stating the vancomycin level for Patient A was high and was not to be given. The drug was due at 8:00 p.m. and had already been administered. The overdose caused kidney failure and Patient A had to have dialysis subsequently.

Here, it must be highlighted how easy it is to forget (remember 'slips and lapses' in Chapter 1).
- ▪ What are the lessons here?
- ▪ What were the mitigating circumstances or contributing factors to the error?
- ▪ What will you do to improve critical communication on the ward?

Nurse

Distraction
Stress
Cognitive overload
Fatigue

Ward clerk

No indication in tone or body language that the information was critical.

It is crucial for healthcare professionals to communicate effectively with each other to ensure safe care. Failure to share critical information can lead to patient harm. Failure to capture or hear information can lead to harm or even death; for example, failure to hear what the patient said about their allergy status may end up causing anaphylaxis.

Verbal and Nonverbal Communication

Although communication can sometimes be regarded as routine, especially repetitive communication, it is a complex phenomenon involving verbal sounds (language) that we make sense of and nonverbal symbols such as body language, tone, pitch, assertiveness and facial expressions.

To achieve this, you must:

- Use terms that people in your care, colleagues and the public can understand
- Take reasonable steps to meet people's language and communication needs, providing, wherever possible, assistance to those who need help to communicate their own or other people's needs
- Use a range of verbal and non-verbal communication methods, and consider cultural sensitivities, to better understand and respond to people's personal and health needs
- Check people's understanding from time to time to keep misunderstanding or mistakes to a minimum
- Be able to communicate clearly and effectively in English (NMC, 2018, p. 10-11).

Verbal Communication

Communication not only includes what is being said but also what is being interpreted; for example, if the surgeon who is performing an open inguinal hernia repair suddenly asks the scrub practitioner for the pool suction in a calm but assertive voice, the scrub practitioner should interpret this as an unexpected critical situation. A potential massive haemorrhage should be the mental image and the scrub practitioner should inform the team to be ready to escalate the protocol. Although the surgeon was calm, the tone of voice and the change in facial expression determined how serious the situation was. The same scenario could be interpreted with less urgency if the tone or change in body language were not noticed. Verbal or spoken communication without nonverbal cues can be misinterpreted or words misunderstood; for example, sarcastic comments can sometimes lead to misinterpretation in culturally diverse teams.

Nonverbal Communication

Do actions speak louder than words? Nonverbal clues and cues can tell a lot about a situation, such as a person's interest in the conversation, and can reinforce verbal conversations, such as looking upset when you say you are upset. For example, landing signal officers on aircraft carriers are trained to not only verbalise orders to the pilot but also to use voice tone and volume to guide the pilot; the pilot is also trained to recognise the urgency in voice tone and volume. In healthcare, these nonverbal clues in commands are essential in critical situations. However, understanding those nonverbal cues depends very much on the experience, familiarity and skills of team members, how many training experiences they have had together as a team and the skills of the leader. The less a team trains together the more chaotic the communication could be—members could speak over each other, give vague instructions and unknowingly vital information is normally lost. Command becomes vague, such as in this example, 'can somebody call blood bank and start the massive haemorrhage protocol?'. Sometimes, everybody will go to the phone or nobody will as they may all assume that somebody else will do it; thus, the blood never arrives which puts the patient at risk. It is widely understood that nonverbal cues in communication play a vital role and indeed can be more important than the words spoken and used; for example, even if the right thing is said, it could go unnoticed if there was no assertiveness in the instruction. In contrast, a situation can be saved even if concerns were not communicated but were recognised through body language or facial expressions. Nevertheless, verbal communication is always a prerequisite.

NONCOMMUNICATION AND COMMUNICATION BREAKDOWN

Can I stay quiet and ignore what I am seeing? The answer is no. In healthcare, you cannot hold your peace. However, communication may break down from time to time for many reasons. Communication is an essential component in healthcare, is the common thread of everything we do and everything depends upon it. Even with communication models, tools to improve communication, such as the situation, background, assessment, recommendation (SBAR) approach or a theatre safety checklist, communication failures still occur. When we see something wrong that is about to happen, it is the duty of the healthcare practitioners to speak up. What if they do speak up and are ignored? How do we manage that situation? Do we receive difficult communication or assertiveness training as part of essential role development? Communication training sessions are an important element of continuing professional development and are essential to prevent and reduce communication errors. Healthcare professionals are bound by the duty of candour.

The professional duty of candour lists the following:

- Tell the patient (or, where appropriate, the patient's advocate, carer or family) when something has gone wrong
- Apologise to the patient (or, where appropriate, the patient's advocate, carer or family)
- Offer an appropriate remedy or support to put matters right (if possible)
- Explain fully to the patient (or, where appropriate, the patient's advocate, carer or family) the short and long term effects of what has happened (NMC & GMC, 2022, p.1). However, healthcare professionals also need training, coaching and ultimately support (Case Study 7.1).

CASE STUDY 7.1

I am a scrub practitioner working in the cardiac surgical team. On one of the days I was scrubbing at the table, I realised after having completed my swab and instruments count that a swab was missing. The surgery was almost ending because the surgeon was closing the layers. On the board it was noted that a swab was used as a pack in the chest wall cavity. I informed the surgeon immediately and informed the team to start a search. We could not find the swab and I asked the surgeon to stop and look for the swab in the chest cavity. He was adamant it was not there, and that it was my fault the swab was lost. My HCA, who is very experienced, tried to tell the surgeon to stop and he retorted that the patient was very ill and needed to be sent to the ITU immediately. I looked at the anaesthetist and he shook his head informing me that he would not challenge the surgeon. I knew I had to escalate this to my matron but it was a weekend and she was not on site. I suggested that we do a CXR before the patient left, per our policy, but the surgeon insisted he was not willing to wait. We compromised and agreed to have the CXR conducted in the ITU.

- The CXR conducted in the ITU an hour later confirmed the swab was in the chest cavity.
- Would graded assertiveness work here?
- Did communication fail or the team fail? Or did both fail?

HOW TO IMPROVE COMMUNICATION AND REDUCE COMMUNICATION ERRORS?

On a day-to-day basis, a healthcare practitioner uses many ways to communicate information to individuals or teams. Some communication may be one-way communication, such as sending an email or informing another individual to go on their break. One-way verbal communication is useful if performed properly; if not adequate instructions are not shared, the message can be lost or ignored.

Example One

Nurse A is speaking to a group of nurses at the desk: 'Can one of you go on break before it gets busy, please (vaguely looking at the team)?'. Then she walks away.

In this type of situation, people may ignore the instruction because it is vague and does not specifically address any single individual. Someone may be thinking that another nurse is not busy or that they have already agreed to their break and so Nurse A could not be addressing them. Although this is a simplistic example, errors or delay in treatment happen because of one-way communication; the individuals or the team do not have the same mental model and assume something else. For example, if the instruction is, 'can somebody brings some Gelofusine for me please?'. Again, who will get the Gelofusine? Will they rush to get it if they do not know that the patient is hypotensive or if the tone of the instruction was flat and not given with assertiveness? Someone could assume that the Gelofusine is just needed for restocking the fluid drawer.

Example Two

Nurse A is speaking to Paul who is at the desk with other nurses: 'Paul (looking at Paul), I need a bag of Volplex solution right now, my patient is hypotensive'. It is very likely that Paul will follow the instruction and bring the fluid immediately.

However, there is a chance that Paul could bring Hartmann's Solution rather than Volplex because there are many variables that could interfere with the communication here (Box 7.2).

BOX 7.2 ■ Variables that Could Interfere with Communication

- Noise can distort a message
- Language or accent barrier
- Expectations
- Past experience
- Mental model
- Prejudice
- Interference or distractions
- Lack of visual cues
- Confirmation bias
- Sounds alike, looks alike (Fig. 7.1)

A very practical way of avoiding the shortcomings of one-way communication is using two-way communication with confirmation—first to confirm the correct information and second to prevent interference or barriers in the communication (Fig. 7.2).

Effective communication is imperative for most nontechnical skills discussed in the different chapters of this book. There are ways that team communication can be improved or made more effective such as team briefings, huddles and debriefing with a structured checklist. Research has demonstrated that these are effective and improve patient safety only if the initiatives are implemented for what they were intended to do.

We can perform debriefings every day and still not learn much because they may be ineffective, not well led or the team members do not engage. Should the team briefs or huddles include staff well-being so that reasonable precautions or adjustments can be made if someone is not well or mentally ready? Can we plan or preempt in the event of an adverse event? For example, who will

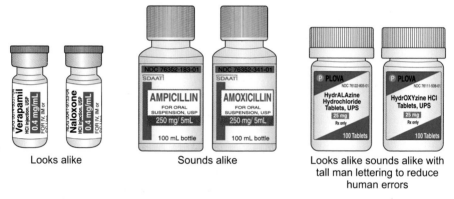

Looks alike   Sounds alike   Looks alike sounds alike with
                                                      tall man lettering to reduce
                                                      human errors

Fig. 7.1   Examples of packaging, vials and bottles that look and sound alike.

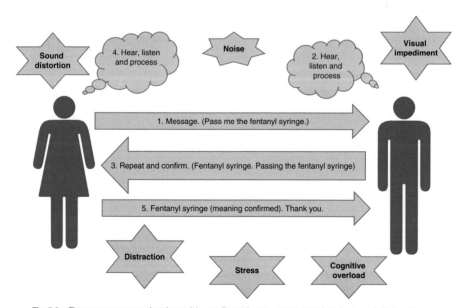

Fig. 7.2   Two-way communication with confirmation to overcome barriers and distractions.

have what responsibilities? In many other areas of healthcare, a team debrief is not part of the daily routine and even the shift handover is mostly regimented to patient care. At the beginning of the shift, are there any reasons why the consultant of the day and other multidisciplinary team members (e.g. physiotherapists and pharmacists) cannot be part of a team brief on the ward? This would surely improve patient safety, and everybody concerned would receive first-hand information which would, in turn, reduce duplication of information as well as risks of communication errors.

Individually, effective communication can be structured by using the SBAR approach, especially in critical situations when the nurse needs to get the attention of the doctor. Sometimes a call-out approach will be effective if someone needs to get the attention of the whole team at the same time or give direct responsibility to a specific person to carry out a specific task so that everybody is aware of who is responsible for what tasks. Here the instruction must be clear, explicit, heard and understood.

In addition, there may be times when an individual or a key member of the team is fixated on a specific task and not listening or sharing the same mental model of the team. This, inevitably, can lead to potential errors and mistakes. Here, assertiveness is required to get the attention of the person, ensure that the person realises the mistake or potential mistake or get the person out of the fixation. The CUS (concern, uncomfortable, stop), DESC (describe, express, suggest, consequences) or PACE (probe, alert, challenge, emergency) techniques are graded assertiveness models that can be helpful to voice and escalate concerns, deescalate difficult situations and stop someone from doing the wrong thing (Table 7.1).

TABLE 7.1 ■ Graded Assertiveness Examples

CUS	DESC	PACE
• Concern: I am concerned you are trying to insert the central line again after two tries. • Uncomfortable: I am uncomfortable because the patient is very upset and does not appear comfortable. • Stop: You need to stop now. I am calling your consultant.	• Describe the specific situation or behaviour and provide concrete evidence: You have tried twice and failed in cannulating the central line. The policy states you can only try twice and then allow someone else to try. • Express how the situation makes you feel and what your concerns are: I am concerned with this situation as I fear you may cause a pneumothorax. The patient is not comfortable and is moving. • Suggest other alternatives and seek agreement: Shall I call your consultant? The consultant is in the department. • Consequences should be stated in terms of the impact on established team goals or patient safety. The goal is to reach consensus: We must stop because the patient is not tolerating this position anymore and the heart rate and breathing have increased.	• Probe: Are you aware that the consent form is not signed? • Alert: Can we check the consent form and assess the situation again? • Challenge: I need you to stop because we are still not sure about the consent form. • Emergency: Stop! We cannot proceed further.

Section Two

ADVANCED COMMUNICATION AND THE PSYCHOSOCIAL ASSESSMENT

As stated in the preceding section, effective communication is 'a two-way process'; the right message is sent and is correctly received and understood by the other person. Effective communication is important when it comes to safety issues in the clinical environment and sensitive engagement between healthcare professionals, patients and their families. Effective communication promotes disclosure of feelings by patients and their families, from which they gain emotional relief—subsequently improving the quality of the interaction as well as patient outcomes such as patient recovery rate, effective pain control, adherence to treatment regimens and psychological functioning. It also creates an environment of trust in which the patient and their family members feel respected and involved.

Poor communication can leave patients feeling anxious, uncertain and generally dissatisfied with their care. Gaps in communication between professionals, caregivers, patients and their families result in decreased quality of care, poor outcomes and dissatisfaction with the healthcare system; these are linked to adverse effects on patient adherence to recommended treatment regimes.

Complaints made by patients frequently focus on perceived failure of communication and an inability to adequately convey a sense of care. Furthermore, the consequences of poor communication can potentially lead to increased stress, lack of job satisfaction and emotional burnout amongst healthcare professionals.

In palliative care and the oncology settings, communication is additionally complicated owing to patients and their families experiencing life-threatening illnesses and bereavement, respectively. In these environments, professionals are often expected to disclose bad news about a life-threatening illness and answer difficult questions related to death and dying that are posed by patients and their families. Many healthcare professionals find this information difficult to communicate, leading to apprehension, avoidance of difficult conversations and misunderstandings among patients, their families and healthcare professionals.

BARRIERS TO COMMUNICATION AMONG PROFESSIONALS, PATIENTS AND THEIR FAMILIES

There are many barriers to establishing effective communication in delicate and complex areas of care, which can arise from the professionals, patients and their family members (Fig. 7.3). Self-awareness, attitudes towards death and dying and the level of facilitative communication skills can affect effective communication. Beliefs and attitudes held by professionals can include assumptions that emotional problems are inevitable and that nothing can be done about them, that talking about concerns that cannot be resolved will falsely raise patient and family expectations and cause more harm than good and that patients will not tolerate the truth and will fall apart. At certain levels within the healthcare hierarchy, some professionals believe that it is not their role to discuss certain things such as particularly sensitive subjects.

Professionals often fear that patients will unleash strong emotions which they will not be able to handle, or will ask difficult or unanswerable questions about diagnosis and dying which the professional may answer incorrectly and get in trouble with their seniors; thus, they stop patients from disclosing their worries by changing the topic or choosing not to initiate the conversation.

Lack of skills in undertaking communication, at what is considered an advanced level, is a common factor of failure in this area. Many professionals do not know how to assess knowledge and perceptions of patients and their families and are not able to integrate medical, psychological, social and spiritual agendas. They lack skills of knowing how to move in and out of strong

FEARS	BELIEFS
Unleashing strong emotions	Emotional problems are inevitable
Upsetting patients/relatives	Not my role
Patient refusing treatment	Talking raises expectations
Difficult questions	Patient will fall apart
Damaging the patient	Will take too long
LACK OF SKILLS	**WORKING ENVIRONMENT**
In assessing knowledge and perceptions	No support or supervision
Integrating medical and psychosocial modes of enquiry	No referral pathway
Handling difficult reactions	Staff conflict
	Lack of time

Fig. 7.3   Barriers to effective communication of healthcare professionals.

emotional expressions of feelings safely and are uncertain how to handle specific communication situations such as breaking bad news.

Lack of adequate support and supervision also contributes to poor communication situations for professionals and, in some cases, organisational culture may promote or inhibit professionals from working to establish therapeutic relationships with patients and their families. The environment in which communication takes place has been identified as a contributing factor of poor communication when institutional demands and heavy workload can limit the time allowed for communication. Nurses tend to use information-giving and practical care strategies to avoid active discussions of patient emotions.

Patient Barriers

Patients also pose barriers when communicating with healthcare professionals. They often lack the appropriate communication skills. For example, they cannot find the right words, do not have sufficient command of the language or are embarrassed about their literacy levels. In many cases, patients do not understand enough to know how to clarify things with the healthcare professional, particularly when the professional has also been posing barriers during the interaction.

The environment, combined with challenging physical barriers such as hearing and vision loss, can also impede good communication interactions with patients. Not having privacy, resulting in embarrassment about revealing intimate concerns, or the presence of protective relatives can also hamper disclosure of concerns by the patient to the healthcare professional. In addition, a patient without a supportive person present can hinder satisfactory communication because the supportive person is often able to ask questions that the patient finds too difficult to address.

Blocking Behaviours

Blocking behaviours by the professional can inhibit patient disclosure of feelings and concerns (Booth et al., 1996; Maguire et al., 1996; Wilkinson, 1991; Wilkinson et al., 2008). There are a multitude of strategies used to block patients from disclosing (Fig. 7.4). Overt blocking is the action of completely changing the topic; a patient may say 'I was very upset about being ill', and the professional responds, 'How's your family?'. Distancing strategies are more subtle and include a change of time frame (e.g. the patient reveals being distressed at a particular point and the professional responds, 'Are you upset now?') or change of person (e.g. the patient responds with 'Was your wife upset?'). Another distancing strategy is the removal of emotion in a response, such as, 'How long were you ill for?'.

Overt blocking
Complete change of topic
Distancing strategies
Change of time frame
Change of person focus
Removal of emotion

Focusing on physical questions
Giving inappropriate information
Focusing on giving advice
Asking closed questions
Asking multiple questions
Asking leading questions
Requesting an explanation
Passing the buck
Defending or justifying
Jollying along
Chit chat

Premature reassurance
Giving advice/information
Normalising
Minimising

Fig. 7.4   Blocking behaviours used by healthcare professionals during communication.

Two of the most common approaches taken by healthcare professionals are focusing on physical symptoms and giving advice. Professionals generally use these tactics because they feel more confident about addressing physical needs and providing advice. In some clinical environments, they are bound by policy to ensure that a patient and their family/support person is given relevant and appropriate information in the form of pamphlets or other healthcare information. Professionals are also generally drawn to focusing on physical symptoms, such as a cough, or some other indication of existing physical symptoms displayed by a patient. They ask questions such as, 'Did you have a lot of symptoms?' and 'What other symptoms have you had?'.

Other examples of blocking behaviour include: defending or justifying an action by a colleague that has distressed the patient of family member in some way, 'I am sure the doctor did not mean to upset you'; giving premature reassurance, 'You will feel better after you have seen the doctor'; premature advice, 'You need to .....' or normalising, 'Everyone gets upset when they are ill'.

Approaches to questioning also contribute to blocking full and open disclosure about concerns from patients to healthcare professionals. An example is the use of closed questions, the responses to which can only be 'yes' or 'no' (e.g. 'Did you tell anyone?'). Only asking for a number or a date is another method. Other types of questioning that can block patient disclosure are asking multiple questions at once (e.g. 'How are you? Is the pain any better?') and asking leading questions (e.g. 'You'll feel better in a minute, won't you?').

FACILITATIVE SKILLS

There are many facilitative techniques that enhance communication (Maguire and Pitceathly, 2002) (Figs 7.5–7.6). Using facilitative communication skills requires an understanding of how communication processes work. Asking open questions is the cornerstone to good communication. Open questions are more complex than simple questions that require a 'yes' or 'no' answer (see Fig. 7.5).

Occasionally, a patient may expand their response; however, using prompts as well as open questions has been found to elicit even more expansive responses from patients and family members. Prompts can include phrases such as, 'tell me more about that' and 'then what happened?'. Gestural prompts are also helpful and can include, nodding, smiling,

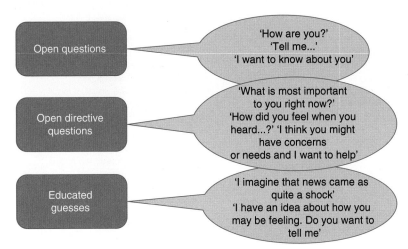

Fig. 7.5   Facilitative skills in communication.

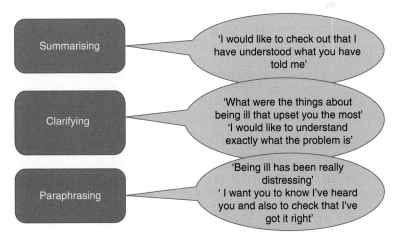

Fig. 7.6   Facilitative skills in simulation.

leaning forward, keeping eye contact (if this is a culturally acceptable approach) and mirroring. Mirroring the body language of the other person makes them feel accepted and creates a bond; mirroring is also similar to reflecting, which involves repeating almost exactly what the speaker said.

Open directive questions are even more complex and enhance the quality of communication encounters. Directive means what something implies and it is direct; using phrases such as, 'can you', 'will you' and 'could you' are not directive, but are requests. A directive question is very specific and starts with phrases such as, 'tell me about', 'please describe', 'share with me', 'help me to understand' and 'what is most important to you right now?' (for further examples, see Fig. 7.5).

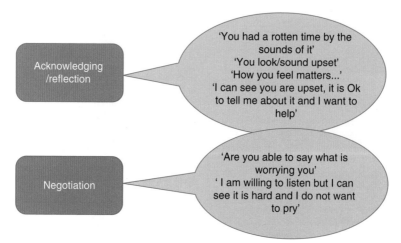

Fig. 7.6 con't   Facilitative skills in simulation.

PICKING UP ON CUES

Picking up on cues is an essential skill when undertaking a psychosocial assessment. Cues are verbal or nonverbal hints which suggest an underlying unpleasant emotion that would need clarifying by a health professional. Facilitative questions linked to a cue increase the probability of further cues and are key to a patient centred consultation (Zimmermann and Del Piccolo, 2007). For example, a patient may use phrases that describe physiological correlates of unpleasant emotional states and say, 'I worry …. about sleep disturbance, loss of libido', or phrases which suggest vague or undefined emotions such as profanities and metaphors, 'it felt odd', 'I cope' and 'it took a while'. These are verbal hints to hidden concerns. These can also include neutral mention of an important/potentially stressful life event, 'I lost my job', 'I had chemotherapy' or mention of a life-threatening diagnosis; these neutral expressions can also be repeated several times in a conversation—thus indicating their importance to the patients. Communication of nonverbal cues can include clear expression of negative or unpleasant emotions (crying) and hints to hidden emotions (sighing, silence after a question, frowning, posture).

LISTENING

For effective communication, listening is an essential skill and involves close attention being paid not only to words but also to emotions of excitement, enthusiasm, interest, anger or fear expressed by the speaker. Listening is multidimensional and complex. It involves cognitive processes (such as attending, understanding and receiving and interpreting messages), affective processes (such as being motivated and stimulated to attend to the message of another person) and behavioural processes (such as responding with verbal and nonverbal feedback) (Bodie and Jones, 2012). Positive outcomes stem from listening and listening-related competencies that lead to more productive interactions, greater relational satisfaction and better healthcare provision. Furthermore, listeners with high people-orientation are nonjudgemental and usually try to find common ground in the communication interaction (Villaume and Bodie, 2007).

There are several recognised types of listening. These include:

- Active listening: the listener listens with all senses, should not interrupt with questions or comments and should give the speakers time to explore their thoughts and feelings.

- Active-empathic listening: requires active, conscious and emotional involvement of a listener attempting to understand what the other person is feeling during an interaction (Bodie, 2011; Gearhart and Bodie, 2011). Comments such as, 'I can see you weren't expecting this', 'This isn't easy to talk about, is it?', 'This must be hard for you' and 'I can see how difficult it is for you', are examples of active-empathic listening.
- Compassionate listening: the primary objective is to recognise the connectedness between those communicating (Rehling, 2008).
- Supportive listening: involves emotional support, is person-centred with immediate nonverbal communication and can include allowing long pauses and silences (Jones, 2011; Bodie and Jones, 2012).

IDENTIFYING THE PATIENT AGENDA WITHIN THE PSYCHOSOCIAL ASSESSMENT

Identifying the patient agenda is a critical feature of an advanced communication. This requires a patient-centred approach that is based on very specific goals: eliciting the patient's perspective on the illness, acknowledging their agenda and concerns, understanding their psychosocial context, negotiating decision-making to reach shared treatment goals based on their values and giving them tailored information effectively. This approach builds on discussions and decisions that involve shared information, compassionate and empowering care provision, sensitivity to patient needs and relationship building. The approach should be jargon free and it is important to give the patients ample time to respond or ask questions. It may be useful to provide simple written instructions, when necessary, and using graphics where possible. Finally, any engagement of a sensitive nature should end with an arrangement to follow up in some way. This could involve making a confirmed date to meet again or a referral to someone else or another service.

EXERCISE 7.1

A woman in her sixties was recently diagnosed with advanced ovarian cancer that has metastasised. She is in an acute hospital ward waiting for treatment. Whilst being attended to by a nurse she asks, 'Am I dying?'.

- What is the cue in this question?
- What type of blocking behaviours might you use to avoid this conversation going any further?
- Why would you use these?
- What facilitative skills would you use?

Use Fig. 7.7 to help you focus on how you would engage with patients and their families when dealing with sensitive and emotional areas.

Conclusion

The paradox of communication is that it something incredibly simple and yet often fails because of communication complexities, ineffective communication or lack of communication. Furthermore, many other nontechnical skills such as situation awareness, teamwork and leadership may fail because of communication. Healthcare professionals must be equipped and trained to become effective at all types and all levels of communication, and its importance must be recognised by the organisations. Formalised communication aids, such as checklist for tasks and procedures, must

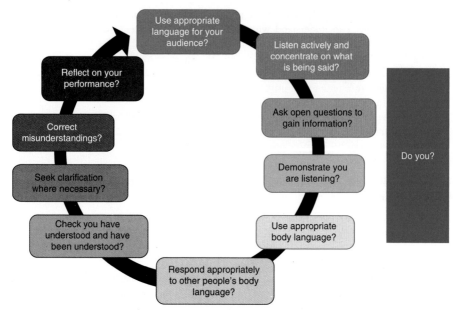

Fig 7.7 Checklist to identify areas for improvement.

become part of our routines as nurses and allied health professionals. Disparities in communication aids or tools that are used, especially on the wards and nonacute areas, must be addressed as failures because these errors can arise everywhere.

Key Points

- Effective communication can be learned, assessed and developed
- Use the two-way communication model and confirm information
- Tools can be used to improve communication
- Lessons should be learned and shared
- Communication is vital for other nontechnical skills

Useful Links

Ausmed, 2019. Communication Skills: A Guide to Practice for Healthcare Professionals 2019. https://www.ausmed.com/cpd/guides/communication-skills.

'Finding the Words' is a workbook developed by the National End of Life Care Programme. London. https://www.slideshare.net/NHSIQlegacy/finding-the-words.

Baile, W.F., 2014. The Complete Guide to Communication Skills in Clinical Practice. https://www.mdanderson.org/documents/education-training/icare/pocketguide-texttabscombined-oct2014final.pdf.

This is a practical guide to gaining skills, strategies and approaches to: breaking bad news; addressing emotions; discussing medical errors; cultural competence; challenging emotional conversations with patients and families; and effective communication in supervision.

References

Bodie, G.D., 2011. The Active-Empathic Listening Scale (AELS): conceptualization and evidence of validity within the interpersonal domain. Commun. Q. 59 (3), 277–295.

Bodie, G.D., Jones, S.M., 2012. The nature of supportive listening II: the role of verbal person centeredness and nonverbal immediacy. West. J. Commun. 76 (3), 250–269.

Booth, K., Maguire, P.M., Butterworth, T., Hillier, V.F., 1996. Perceived professional support and the use of blocking behaviours by hospice nurses. J. Adv. Nurs. 24 (3), 522–527.

Flin, R., O'Connor, P., Crichton, M., 2008. Safety at the Sharp End: A Guide to Non-technical Skills. Ashgate Publishing Company, Burlington.

Gearhart, C.C., Bodie, G.D., 2011. Active-empathic listening as a general social skill: evidence from bivariate and canonical correlations. Commun. Rep. 24 (2), 86–98.

Ives, C., Hillier, S., 2015. Human factors in healthcare common terms. In: Clinical Human Factors Group. Working with Clinical Professionals and Managers to Make Healthcare Safer. https://www.chfg.org. (Accessed 7 April 2022).

Jones, S.M., 2011. Supportive listening. Int. J. List. 25 (1–2), 85–103.

Maguire, P., Booth, K., Elliot, C., Jones, B., 1996. Helping health professionals involved in cancer care acquire key interviewing skills – the impact of workshops. Eur. J. Cancer 32A (9), 1486–1489.

Maguire, P., Pitceathly, C., 2002. Key communication skills and how to acquire them. BMJ 325 (7366), 697–700.

Nursing and Midwifery Council, 2018. The Code. https://www.nmc.org.uk/standards/code/. (Accessed 7 April 2023).

Nursing and Midwifery Council & General Medical Council, 2022. The professional duty of candour. https://www.nmc.org.uk/standards/guidance/the-professional-duty-of-candour/read-the-professional-duty-of-candour/.

Parliamentary and Health Service Ombudsman, 2019-20. Complaints about the NHS in England. Quarter 1 2019-20. https://www.ombudsman.org.uk/sites/default/files/Complaints_about_the_NHS_in_England_Quarter_1_2019-20.pdf. (Accessed 5 March 2022).

Rehling, D.L., 2008. Compassionate listening: a framework for listening to the seriously ill. Int. J. List. 22 (1), 83–89.

Villaume, W.A., Bodie, G.D., 2007. Discovering the listener within us: the impact of trait-like personality variables and communicator styles on preferences for listening style. Int. J. List. 21 (2), 102–123.

Wilkinson, S., 1991. Factors which influence how nurses communicate with cancer patients. J. Adv. Nurs. 16 (6), 677–688.

Wilkinson, S., Perry, R., Blanchard, K., Linsell, L., 2008. Effectiveness of a three-day communication skills course in changing nurses' communication skills with cancer/palliative care patients: a randomised controlled trial. Palliat. Med. 22 (4), 365–375.

Zimmermann, C., Del Piccolo, L., Finset, A., 2007. Cues and concerns by patients in medical consultations: a literature review. Psychol. Bull. 133 (3), 438–463.

CHAPTER 8

Situational Awareness and Decision-Making

Lianne McInally

Introduction

Healthcare is a complex system. On a day-to-day basis, there are many situations and decisions that rely on multiple factors. Sometimes these situations and decisions result in high quality care for the individual; however, other times they result in missed care or poor outcomes from the care delivered. Nurses and other healthcare professionals play a critical role in demonstrating vigilance in healthcare, and what they do or fail to do is directly related to patient outcomes (Fore and Sculli, 2013).

Elaine Bromiley was a loving wife and mother. She went to hospital in 2005 for a routine sinus operation. Unfortunately, she died during the operation. Her husband Martin Bromiley was an airline pilot who understood the application of human factors in the airline industry. As a result of her death, he formed the charity Clinical Human Factors Group (CHFG) to integrate human factors in healthcare. He wrote:

> 'In 2005, my late wife died as a direct result of medical errors during a routine operation. A subsequent independent review identified that a well-equipped operating theatre and a team of clinicians—all technically skilled—had failed to respond appropriately to an unanticipated emergency.
> They failed to follow protocols, use equipment properly, maintain situational awareness, prioritise and make decisions appropriately.
> Leadership was confused, communication problems arose despite attempts to speak up by the team and any benefit of the team skills and awareness present was lost.
> In short, human factors, not technical inability, led to my late wife's death'.
> **Martin Bromiley (Bromiley, 2020)**

On that day in 2005, no one came to work with the intention of causing harm to a patient—in this case Elaine Bromiley. On the contrary, all the individuals probably were there because they care. An autonomous 1:1 patient and healthcare professional relationship is highlighted (Babiker et al., 2014) as being important, particularly in nursing, dentistry and medicine. Situational awareness and decision-making are skills that nurses and other healthcare professionals need to understand in order to provide safe, person-centred care.

What Is Situational Awareness?

Situational awareness is defined as an individual, team or organisation having an understanding of what is happening around them and what could happen in the future (Endsley and SA Technologies, 2016; Gonzalez and Wimisberg, 2007; McIntosh, 2018). It plays a key role in task performance and has been linked to a number of industries such as airlines, military, train line, maritime and football strategy (Chavin et al., 2008; Gonzalez and Wimisberg, 2007; Marcus et al., 2020; McIntosh, 2018; Stanton et al., 2001). The concept of situational awareness was originally applied to gaining awareness of the enemy during World War I (Gilson, 1995) and more recently the concept has been applied to healthcare.

Situational awareness supports clinical reasoning. Clinical reasoning ability requires the recognition and incorporation of multiple individual aspects of a patient to enable the best treatment option in any clinical setting (Fischer et al., 2017). Situational awareness in healthcare has been found to significantly correlate with the quality of care and treatment delivered to patients.

For example, a doctor or nurse identifies a change in the condition of a patient, understands this is a bad sign and knows that in half an hour the patient will be in the danger zone and action should be taken now; thus, patient deterioration was detected (Clinical Human Factors Group, 2015).

An everyday example of situational awareness is driving a vehicle. This requires a constant awareness of what is happening on the road, anticipating how an accident may happen and taking action to avoid one. For example, before turning right the driver looks in mirror, checks the cars behind, signals, assesses the speed of oncoming cars and waits until it is safe to turn (Clinical Human Factors Group, 2015).

Consequences of Poor Situational Awareness

When people are required to make critical choices, sometimes at fast pace, the vast majority of errors that occur are a direct result of situational awareness (SA Technologies, 2021). These results can be catastrophic, costing substantial amounts of money, huge inconvenience to people or, most importantly, loss of lives.

For example, in aviation, 583 people lost their lives in the 1977 Tenerife Airport disaster, which occurred due to a collision between two planes. Apparently, the disaster was a direct result of lack of situational awareness; a plane was mistakenly cleared for take-off. The pilot and copilot of the KLM flight realised it was too late when they caught sight of the PanAm flight through the fog (Green et al., 2017).

In healthcare, poor situational awareness can result in serious compromise to patient safety if it is not recognised by an individual or the team (Integrated Human Factors, 2022). Elaine Bromiley has become associated with one of the most significant events in healthcare that can be attributed to situational awareness. Unfortunately, this is not an isolated incident. Another patient, Felicity, had right-sided bleeding in her brain as a result of a significant medication error (Integrated Human Factors, 2022). She was 4 years old and had been admitted to the cardiology ward owing to fluid in her lungs. Felicity was prescribed 1520 units of dalteparin medication twice daily. However, when the dose was entered into the electronic prescribing information technology

(IT) system, the prescriber did not make the necessary manual alteration to the dose within the system to reflect her age and weight. The dalteparin was then inadvertently prescribed at a dose of 15,200 units twice daily. This meant Felicity received 15,200 units of dalteparin (10 times the dose intended) on five occasions over one weekend. A subsequent computed tomography (CT) scan showed that Felicity had a new right-sided bleed in the brain (Healthcare Safety Investigation Branch, 2022).

The process for checking medication for Felicity was variable and multiple cues influenced whether staff considered doses to be correct (Healthcare Safety Investigation Branch, 2022). There were five occasions over one weekend where there was an opportunity for someone to have realised the error, but no one did. If we assume that there could have been more than one individual responsible for the administration of the medicine, then there were also multiple opportunities for more than one person to identify the error. Studies have found that nurses and other healthcare professionals are able to identify medication errors but are reluctant to report them. Fear of the consequences is the main reason given for not reporting medication errors (Dirik et al., 2019). In addition, nurses need to cope with time pressures, completing work quickly and the constant flow of information with which they are bombarded. Failure to juggle everything can lead to low situational awareness (Chu, 2016). In the case of Felicity, all these factors could have impacted her outcome.

Accurate and safe medication administration depends on nurses' pharmacologic knowledge and decision-making and critical thinking skills (Dirik et al., 2019). The error happened over a weekend and there could have been limited staffing. Lack of adequate staffing increases workload and fatigue, which negatively affect nurses' and other healthcare professionals' work performance related to drug administration (Dirik et al., 2019). This could be attributed to the medication error. In addition, interruptions during medication dispensing have also been highlighted to contribute to medication errors (Sitterding et al., 2014). Again, these factors may have impacted the ability for nurses and other healthcare professionals to recognise the error.

Poor situational awareness is often displayed in other high-risk areas of inpatient care, such as emergency departments, operating theatres, obstetrics and intensive care units (ICUs). Emergency departments are notoriously known for their poor situational awareness due to the unpredictable, dynamic and often chaotic environment with poor information (Lowe et al., 2016). People visit emergency departments when they have an acute illness that can deteriorate quickly. There can be multiple emergency admissions all at once and often previous medical information is not available. Operating theatres can present similar challenges, particularly in emergency situations; 50% of identified adverse events that occurred in the operating theatre were preventable (Lowe et al., 2016). Likewise, 62% of obstetrics cases that required critical incident review for adverse events were caused by cognitive errors due to a lack of situational awareness and inappropriate decision-making that could have been prevented (Hinshaw, 2016).

A study of ICU team members found that individuals had conflicting anticipations as to whether patients would deteriorate within 48 hours. Staggeringly, this effect was found for 50% of the patients in the ICU and it was attributed to healthcare team members' situational awareness (Gillespie et al., 2013). More recently, given the coronavirus disease 2019 (COVID-19) pandemic and significant pressures in the ICU, this figure could potentially be higher. ICU capacity was increased to help cope with the demand of the pandemic. Healthcare staff were redeployed to support ICU teams. The initial surge was complex not only because of the repeated changes in clinical protocols and exponential number of patients with severe COVID-19 pneumonia but also because of the unparalleled degree of uncertainty surrounding the disease trajectory (Kentish-Barnes et al., 2021). All these factors combined may have impacted staff situational awareness.

Situational awareness in healthcare can occur at micro (individual), meso (team) or macro (organisational) levels. It cannot only be attributed to inpatient care. Approximately 33% of lung and colorectal cancer diagnostic errors in primary care were found to be attributed to situational awareness at both individual and team levels (Singh et al., 2012). A study of patient safety skills in primary care identified that general practitioners (GPs) identified situational awareness as an important factor in the community (Ahmed et al., 2014). For primary care physicians, it plays an important role in providing proactive care for people with complex health conditions (Berkeley Institute for Data Science, 2022). In addition, primary care nurses must have an understanding of the needs of patients, family members, physicians and healthcare environments (Davis, 2016); situational awareness plays an important role in enabling nurses to provide high-quality, person-centred care.

Situational awareness is important at the organisational level. Following Hurricane Rita, the Gulf Coast evacuation plans of acute hospitals were systematically reviewed. Particular attention was given to individual hospital responses. Poor decision-making and response was attributed to lack of situational awareness. Seven hospital evacuation plans for Hurricane Rita were analysed. The review concluded that successful evacuation was dependent on community wide situational awareness (Downey et al., 2013). The hospital that activated their plan quickest was at the heart of Hurricane Rita. The second hospital to activate their plan was the hospital that had been closest to a previous event, Hurricane Katrina. The study concluded that situational awareness impacted the speed at which each hospital enacted its plan.

Situational awareness was also influential in the population response to the H1N1 and COVID-19 pandemics. A study of health protective behaviours during the H1N1 pandemic found that there was a correlation between situational awareness and response to the pandemic; it was associated with the impact on protective behaviours. Those with poor situational awareness were more unlikely to adhere to protective awareness. Epidemic situational awareness is probably derived from multiple sources including formally announced public information, news items, government press releases and informal sources such as social media (Liao et al., 2010). Social distancing was found to be influenced by situational awareness gained from news and other media sources (Qazi et al., 2020). The more media-aware individuals were, the more likely they were to adhere to safe distancing. Public Health England (2021) used a daily situational awareness report as part of the COVID-19 pandemic response. This daily report maintained the visibility of the pandemic and enabled the public in the United Kingdom to visibly see the size and scale of the pandemic—based on the theory that more people would adhere to health protective behaviours as a result.

There has been much debate about government response to the COVID-19 pandemic during the initial wave. In the United Kingdom, Professor Edmunds, who was part of the government Scientific Advisory Group for Emergencies (SAGE), attributed poor situational awareness to the delay of lockdown measures in the United Kingdom. He stated, 'I think the data that we were dealing with in the early part of March and our situational awareness was really quite poor' (BBC News, 2020). There is increasing opinion that this may have cost lives during the first wave of the pandemic. An independent enquiry is ongoing.

Three Levels of Situational Awareness and How They Relate to Healthcare

Over the last 25 years, Mica Endsley has been the leading researcher of situational awareness and has proposed a three level framework (Endsley, 2016):

- Level one: Perception; knowing that something has occurred within the elements of the environment.
- Level two: Comprehension; what does the status of what has happened indicate?
- Level three: Projection; how will what has happened project into the future?

These three levels are interdependent on one another and ultimately affect the decision-making of individuals and outcomes of a situation (Fig. 8.1).

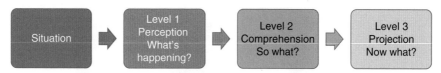

Fig. 8.1 Three levels of situational awareness.

LEVEL ONE: PERCEPTION

Perception is defined an awareness of things around you and is often linked to our senses—particularly sight and hearing (Cambridge Dictionary, 2021). It is the ability to interpret what is happening in a particular situation or task. Perception of critical information or data is necessary to ensure good situational awareness. Perception allows an individual to make decisions based on the way they process that information. This is considered to be one of the main factors that have contributed to accidents in aviation as well as healthcare. An analysis of anaesthesia incidents revealed that 38% of these were a direct result of level one perception errors (Schulz et al., 2016). However, Endsley and Jones (1996) found that failure to perceive a situation could account for as much as 76% of errors.

Think of your own situational awareness. The following are some key questions to consider:
- Do we always see what we think we see?
- Do we have sufficient knowledge to understand what is going on around us?
- Could our knowledge be influenced by the views of others or our previous experiences?
- Does the time we have allow us to have an accurate enough perception of the situation?

The reason so many incidents, accidents, errors may be attributed to perception is that it is individualised. The most famous example of perception are the Gestalt figure-ground pictures (Gleitman et al., 2010)—people may see a vase/chess piece or two faces (Fig. 8.2). These pictures highlight that environmental factors, such as the depth of the black and white images or the way the images are imposed black on white or white on black, have an impact on the way an individual perceives them.

Perception is also linked to a phenomenon called inattentional blindness. Researchers have shown that people often miss the occurrence of an unexpected yet salient event if they are engaged in a different task. This is known as inattentional blindness. A group of 24 radiologists were asked to perform a familiar lung-nodule detection task. A gorilla, 48 times the size of the average nodule, was inserted in the last case that was presented; 83% of the radiologists did not see the gorilla. Eye tracking revealed that the majority of those who missed the gorilla looked directly at its location. Thus, even experts are vulnerable to inattentional blindness. Fig. 8.3 outlines the X-ray that was shown to these radiologists (Drew et al., 2013); can you find the gorilla?

Another example of inattentional blindness can be found online in the Basketball Gorilla Trick (Simons, 2012). Based on work of Simons and Chabris (1999), who highlighted that we perceive and remember only the objects (or events) that have our focused attention, participants were asked to watch a basketball video and count how many times the ball is passed between players. Whilst doing so, a person dressed as a gorilla walked into the middle of the scene. When participants were asked at the end if they noticed the gorilla, very few reported they had. This is because their focus was in attending to the task rather than on the rest of the surroundings.

Challenges with situational awareness arise from being unable to perceive a situation as a result of multiple factors (Gleitman, 2010):
- Information is not available: This can be due to the system or design factors, failures communicating information and failures of individuals or teams to perform a required task. For example, a patient admitted to the emergency department has a lack of medical history. This information is either not available or is available on a different system. Another clinical

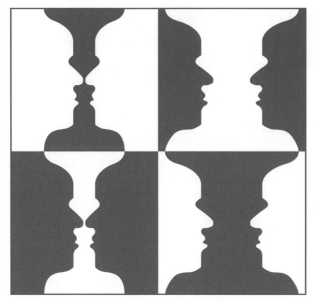

Fig. 8.2   Gestalt figure–ground pictures. (Gleitman et al. 2010.)

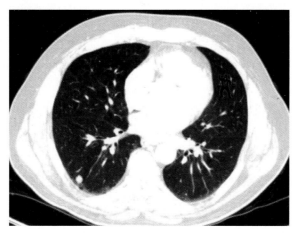

Fig. 8.3   X-ray.

example is when a pulmonary angiogram was performed on a patient with an elevated creatinine level but the radiologist was unaware that the patient was experiencing renal failure (Murphy et al., 2010).

■ Information is difficult to detect: This can be due to environment designs such as poor signage, making it difficult to perceive what is happening, poor working conditions, noise that causes a distraction, transitions of care/handover information and staff turnover/absence/agency; for example, a person does not observe the information which leads to missed care (Suhonen and Scott, 2018). This can happen because of not scanning for all the correct information, lack of attention because of task-related distractions, workload and individual experience such as being new to a work area and unfamiliarity with systems and processes.

- Misperception: Owing to previous experiences, individuals may misperceive a situation and assume that the circumstances are the same as previous situations. This commonly happens when two simultaneous events occur as per a person's expectations. The person has subconsciously created a mental model for those events and assumes that the outcomes will be the same again (Besnard et al., 2004). For example, a clinician assesses a person who smells of alcohol and has reduced level of consciousness. The clinician, if inexperienced, may conclude this is the result of alcohol ingestion and not consider other causes such as head injury (Besnard et al., 2004). Misperception can also happen during surgical procedures. A study on a bile duct surgery found that 97% of errors were caused from misperception by the surgeons. They either misperceived that the common duct (or right hepatic duct) was the cystic duct, which was followed by deliberately cutting the misidentified duct, or made an error in dissecting the triangle of Calot unintentionally too close to the bordering common hepatic or right hepatic duct (Way et al., 2003).

- Memory error: This can be due to distractions in routine or high workloads and cognitive overload; for example, someone makes a medication error such as forgetting to give a patient a medication dose. Medication errors may occur during any phase of the medication process: prescribing, transcribing, dispensing, administering, monitoring and reporting (Chu, 2016). Distractions are a leading cause of pharmacy errors when dispensing medicine to patients (Way et al., 2003). Distractions can occur when a person is interrupted during a task. It is estimated that healthcare staff are interrupted every 2 minutes (Chu, 2016). Interruptions can be due to patients requiring immediate assistance or relatives or staff members requiring attention. When the person dispensing the medication returns to the task, they may miss a patient or perceive that they have already attended to a task.

Additionally, in primary care, diagnostic errors or delays have been attributed to memory errors. One primary care physician admitted not remembering to order a colonoscopy test for a person with abnormal blood results (Singh et al., 2012).

Chronic excessive workload is a key driver for burnout within healthcare and this has a significant role in perception and situational awareness (Reader et al., 2016). Fig. 8.4 highlights the relationship between the increasing resource demands of the task (horizontal axis) versus the physiological activation level (right vertical axis) and resultant task performance (left vertical axis). There is an optimum level wherein the combination of all these factors will lead to an individual being able to perform well.

Information processing also plays a part in perception. The cognitive load theory (Sweller, 1988) suggests that the amount of information we are able to process and remember is limited by our working memory. In order to remember information over a longer time period, the information must be processed from working memory to long-term memory. Working memory supports many kinds of mental abilities. It allows an individual to retain multiple pieces of information for use in the moment, which is essential for activities ranging from reading and having a conversation to learning new concepts and making decisions between different options (Psychology Today, 2022). The average human can hold seven items in their working memory (plus or minus two) (InnerDrive, 2022; The Human Memory, 2022). However, the amount of information a person can retain is influenced by a number of factors. Cognitive load plays a significant role in working memory and the ability of an individual to process information—thus impacting perception. There are three distinct, interlinked elements in cognitive load: intrinsic, extraneous and germane (InnerDrive, 2022; Mcdreeamie-musings, 2019; Psychology Today, 2022; Sweller, 1988; The Human Memory, 2022; van Merriënboer and Sweller, 2010).

- Intrinsic load is the difficulty and detail of the task/information itself. This can be influenced by prior knowledge of the topic and is dependent on the complexity of the new information.

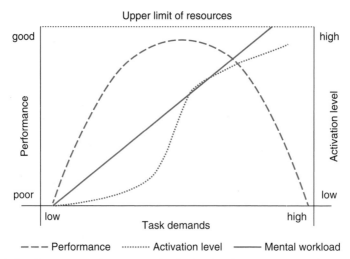

Fig. 8.4 Relationship among performance, activation level and mental workload. (Young et al. 2015.)

- Extraneous load is generated by the way the task/information is presented. If the extraneous load is too high, it distracts working memory from processing information.
- Germane load is the deep processing of information to create permanent storage of knowledge, and integrating it with previous learning.

Cognitive overload occurs when the cognitive load outweighs the processing capacity. This can happen for a number of reasons (InnerDrive, 2022):

- The task is taking too long.
- The task is too difficult.
- There are too many choices.
- Too much information is presented all at once.

Cognitive overload can lead to an individual feeling overwhelmed, disengaged and intimidated, and affects the ability to be productive.

Cognitive balance occurs when there is sufficient processing capacity available for the required load. Fig. 8.5 outlines how balancing cognitive load improves processing capacity and ensures the productivity of an individual.

Perception can be affected by other factors that may impact performance ability during a work day. Errors are more likely to occur under certain circumstances (Health and Safety Executive, 1999), including:

- Work environment stressors: extremes of heat, humidity, noise, vibration, poor lighting and restricted workspace.
- Extreme task demands: high workload, tasks demanding high levels of alertness, very monotonous and repetitive jobs and situations with many distractions and interruptions.
- Social and organisational stressors: insufficient staff levels, inflexible or over demanding work schedules, conflicts with work colleagues, peer pressure and conflicting attitudes concerning health and safety.
- Individual stressors: inadequate training and experience, high fatigue levels, reduced alertness, family problems, ill health and misuse of alcohol and drugs.
- Equipment stressors: poorly designed displays and controls and inaccurate and confusing instructions and procedures.

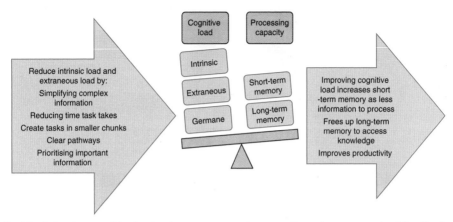

Fig. 8.5 Balancing cognitive load to improve processing capacity and ensure productivity. (Sweller, 1988; Psychology Today, 2022; InnerDrive, 2022; The Human Memory, 2022; Mcdreeamie-musings, 2019; van Merriënboer and Sweller, 2010.)

Maslow's hierarchy of needs (Maslow, 1943, 1954) indicates that the most basic human need is physiological (food, water, warmth, rest) (Fig. 8.6). According to this hierarchy, our basic needs must be met for us to function. If we are not able to meet the basic needs, then this has a direct impact on psychological needs and our ability to achieve our potential. Many of the factors that are referenced to cause errors can be linked to the basic physiological, safety and security needs of this hierarchy.

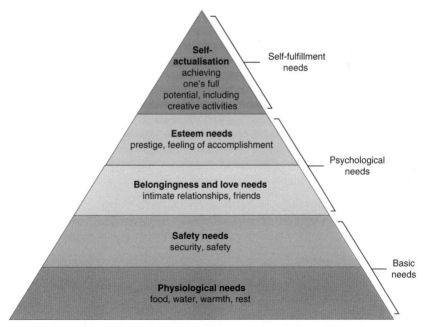

Fig. 8.6 Maslow's hierarchy of needs. (Maslow, 1943, 1954)

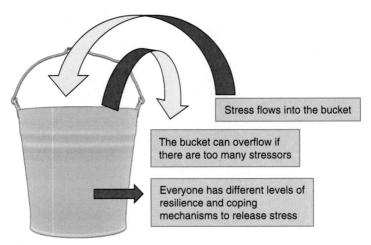

Stress flows into the bucket

The bucket can overflow if there are too many stressors

Everyone has different levels of resilience and coping mechanisms to release stress

Fig. 8.7 **The model of the stress and vulnerability bucket.** (Brabban et al., 2002.)

In healthcare, the demands and complexity of workload and patient encounters mean that many staff members do not have their basic needs met during their working day. A staff survey found that over two-thirds of nurses (70%) skipped some or all their breaks during their shift (UNISON, 2015). One respondent said, 'I'm always exhausted, dehydrated and hungry when I finish my shift'. This has a direct impact on the perception of individuals, either consciously or subconsciously, because their ability to process and perceive information may be distorted by the fact that they have not fulfilled their basic human needs. Consequently, the repeated cycle of being unable to meet basic human needs can lead to higher stress levels.

The model of the stress and vulnerability bucket (Brabban and Turkington, 2002) is comparative to the concept of balancing cognitive loading and it explains how a person's resilience in handling situations can be impacted by the amount of stressors that person is carrying in their bucket (Fig. 8.7). Many people have a workplace bucket and a home bucket. Similar to cognitive loading, if the buckets are not balanced, then this can cause coping ability issues for the individual. Stress accounted for a loss of 511,000 days to healthcare owing to sick leave taken by staff (Brennan et al., 2020).

Stress can have a direct impact on perception because the amount of stress may affect a person's level of mental abstraction when processing information (Brennan et al., 2020). It is important to recognise stress and support people to release their stress and prevent their bucket from overflowing.

Ensuring that there is a correct balance of stressors and cognitive load supports healthcare staff so that they can confidently move from level one (perception) to level two (comprehension).

LEVEL TWO: COMPREHENSION

Comprehension has been described by Endsley (2016) as the 'so what' of situational awareness—understanding the meaning of the information. This is the ability of the individual to interpret the information they have and make decisions based on their understanding of this information.

Challenges with situational awareness arise from being unable to comprehend a situation due to several factors (Stanton et al., 2001):
- Lack of or an incomplete mental model: A mental model is a personal explanation of an individual's thought process of how something works. Lack of a mental model or an incomplete mental model leads to being unable to fully comprehend a situation.

- Use of an incorrect mental model: A person may use the wrong mental model owing to an assumption made about a situation. This may also be due to lack of situational experience. A fight or flight response can impact the use of an incorrect mental model. Given the nature of healthcare, there are multiple situations when staff may elicit a fight or flight response that may also have an immediate and sustained impact on cognition (Civil Aviation Authority, 2014).
- Overreliance on default models: A person may have a mental model for a particular situation and use it time and time again. However, this default model may not be correct in some situations.

Comprehension can be affected by the skill level of an individual. This is because comprehension requires an individual to assess the integrity and accuracy of data and their relevance to a situation (Fischer et al., 2017). It is always more difficult to achieve a skilled task when a person starts to learn it; however, with repeated practice, the skill becomes easier to implement. This applies to complex skills more than it does to simple skills. Early studies of situational awareness found that novice pilots had a lower level of level two situational awareness than did expert pilots (Civil Aviation Authority, 2014). This is similar to healthcare—junior trainees may have satisfactory situational awareness at level one but might not comprehend all the information, and therefore have lower level two situational awareness (Green et al., 2017). Trainees and experienced staff are both vulnerable to lack of situational awareness for differing reasons (Hinshaw, 2016); this is shown in the previous example where experienced radiographers failed to spot the gorilla on an X-ray (Fig. 8.3). Tunnel vision is reported to be one of the most significant reasons why people are unable to comprehend information (Brennan et al., 2020; Green et al., 2017). A healthcare professional experiencing tunnel vision is focused on one single aspect of patient care or they may have an overreliance on a particular mental model. Although there may be a perfectly valid reason to focus on one particular task, this reduced awareness to comprehend a situation can be detrimental to safety.

LEVEL THREE: PROJECTION

Projection is the ability to understand how the information in the current situation may impact the immediate future. At this level, a person can forecast future events and dynamics. People who have a high level of situational awareness display this characteristic. The accuracy of projection is dependent on the precision gained in levels one and two (Green et al., 2017).

Similar to level two, a lack of or an incomplete mental model can impact level three (projection). In addition, challenges can occur when a person overprojects the situation based on current trends (Stanton et al., 2001).

Situational awareness is a dynamic process and the progression from level one to level three is not linear. 'A person who understands the current situation has better situational awareness than one who can read the data on a screen but does not know what it means. Similarly, a person who can project the likely future events and states of the system and environment has better situational awareness than one who cannot' (Endsley, 2015).

Situational Awareness and Its Relationship to Healthcare

Fig. 8.8 outlines the relationship between situational awareness and healthcare. When a patient presents as unwell, it is a dynamic situation. What is happening at level one may change over time and impact the 'so what' and 'now what' factors of the situation. Information is passed between the levels, and how this is processed and actioned at each level will impact outcomes.

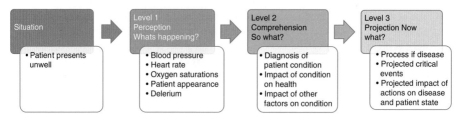

Fig. 8.8   Situational awareness and its relationship to healthcare.

WHAT DOES PERCEPTION LOOK LIKE IN HEALTHCARE?

A nurse and other healthcare professional have to perceive various pieces of information about a patient in their care and understand what is happening to the patient. These may be based on information that is known about medical history, medications being taken and vital signs such as blood pressure, heart rate and oxygen levels. They may also be involved in recognising improvement or deterioration in a patient over time and the rate at which that change happens. They may be based on speech, cognitive ability, mobility and function of a patient. They may also have to observe how the patient looks or presents.

WHAT DOES COMPREHENSION LOOK LIKE IN HEALTHCARE?

A nurse and other healthcare professionals have to comprehend how the information they have perceived relates to a patient's current health status. They must understand what this means for the patient and what action they will need to take. They may have to use the information perceived to diagnose a patient's condition. They have to understand what the effect of the current condition is and what impact it has on the health and social care of a patient. They are also required to understand the impact of other factors such as introducing a treatment, intervention and the current environment in which the treatment is being administered.

WHAT DOES PROJECTION LOOK LIKE IN HEALTHCARE?

A nurse and other healthcare professionals have to project how the information they have perceived and comprehended relates to a patient's future health status. What is the prognosis for a diagnosis? What is predicted to happen to a patient?

The outcomes of a situation will be dependent on all the variables comprising perception, comprehension and projection.

Development of Situational Awareness from Novice to Expert

Situational awareness is linked to the skill level of a person (Stanton et al., 2001). Experts have a higher level of skill and situational awareness than does a novice, because they know more, their knowledge is better organised and integrated, they have better strategies for accessing knowledge and using it, they are self-regulated and have different motivations (Didau, 2017). A fun example of this journey has been adapted from the Star Wars movies; the journey to become a Jedi Knight starts visually with Luke Skywalker as a novice and is completed with the master Yoda (Fig. 8.9).

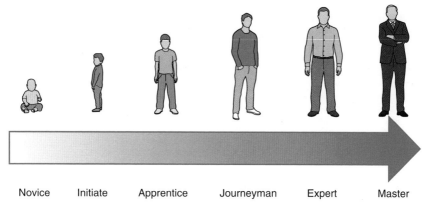

Novice   Initiate   Apprentice   Journeyman   Expert   Master

Fig. 8.9 The novice to expert journey. (Didau, 2017.)

Another example of the novice to expert journey is driving a vehicle. Novice learners have been found to perform significantly worse than experienced drivers when required to identify and locate a hazard and predict what will happen next (Gugliotta et al., 2017). Statistics also suggest that younger, newly qualified drivers are more likely to have an accident because they do not have the experience of driving in various situations and are more likely to take risks (UK Parliament House of Commons Transport Committee, 2021).

Similar results have been observed in healthcare; nursing students have been found to demonstrate situational awareness levels one through three but their awareness varies (Tower et al., 2019). The novice nurse who is at the beginning of training is likely to have a task list and focus on this, whereas the expert nurse would focus on the whole picture (Nursing Theory, 2020). Benner (2001) highlighted five stages of clinical competence in nursing, which are outlined in Table 8.1 (Nursing Theory, 2020).

Team Versus Individual Situational Awareness

Often in healthcare, teams work together on tasks towards a common end goal that often involves a patient; therefore, it is important that individual members not only have good situational awareness but also shared situational awareness (Gillespie et al., 2013).

A healthcare team consists of a range of staff who have different experiences and skill levels, from novice to expert; they have different professions such as nurse, doctor, occupational therapist or physiotherapist. Support staff also have different skill levels. There is a risk of performance breakdown in teams when the members are not able to anticipate the help needed because decisions are made based on the information gained from all team members in order to establish an action plan (Green et al., 2017). An individual may assume that their level one perception and level two comprehension of information are the same as that of everyone else in the team, and therefore their level three projection would also be the same.

Failure to covey time-critical information during surgery diminishes a team member's perceptions of the dynamic information relevant to their tasks and compromises team-shared situational awareness (Gillespie et al., 2013; Hinshaw, 2016). Team situational awareness played a significant role in the errors that lead to the death of Elaine Bromiley, described in the introduction of this chapter.

Although teams working together can potentially compromise safety, teams are found to be more robust in enhancing situational awareness and facing unexpected events or emergencies than

TABLE 8.1 ■ Stages of Clinical Competence in Nursing (Nursing Theory, 2020)

Stage 1: Novice	Stage 2: Advanced Beginner	Stage 3: Competent	Stage 4: Proficient	Stage 5: Expert
For nursing students in their first year of clinical education, behaviour in the clinical setting is very limited and inflexible. Novices have a very limited ability to predict what might happen in a particular patient situation. Signs and symptoms, such as change in mental status, can only be recognised after a novice nurse has had experience with patients with similar symptoms.	New graduates in their first jobs. These nurses have had more experiences that enable them to recognise recurrent, meaningful components of a situation. They have the knowledge and the know-how but not enough in-depth experience.	These nurses lack the speed and flexibility of proficient nurses, but they have some mastery and can rely on advance planning and organisational skills. Competent nurses recognise patterns and the nature of clinical situations more quickly and accurately than do advanced beginners.	At this level, nurses are capable of seeing situations as 'wholes' rather than 'parts'. Proficient nurses have learned from experience what events typically occur and are able to modify plans in response to different events.	Nurses who are able to recognise demands and resources in situations and attain their goals. These nurses know what needs to be done. They no longer rely solely on rules to guide their actions under certain situations. They have an intuitive grasp of the situation based on their deep knowledge and experience. Their focus is on the most relevant problems and not irrelevant ones. Analytical tools are used only when they have no experience with an event or when events do not occur as expected.

are individuals (Hinshaw, 2016; She and Li, 2017). Communication and team cognition are key to team situational awareness (Pollack et al., 2020). In addition, creating an environment where an individual or team are encouraged to do the right thing at the right time for the right person leads to good situational awareness.

Teams can exist within an organisation and across organisations. Having situational awareness across organisational teams has been attributed to decision-making during the H1N1 outbreak (Liao et al., 2010) and hospital evacuations due to hurricanes in the United States of America (Downey et al., 2013). Situational awareness for outbreaks and hurricanes requires real-time data. When teams across organisations rely on perceptual information that is likely acquired from surveillance systems designed to look for large scale events, subtle changes may be more difficult to perceive across organisations. The added challenge is that information may be required from a variety of sources.

What Is the Relevance of Situational Awareness and Decision-making in Healthcare?

To achieve situational awareness, you require appropriate current information and the correct perception of the current information to enable you to make good decisions. Fig. 8.10 shows the integration of situational awareness with decisions and actions. This process is dynamic; often there are multiple sources of information that require decisions and actions.

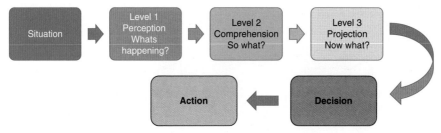

Fig. 8.10 Integration of situational awareness with decisions and actions.

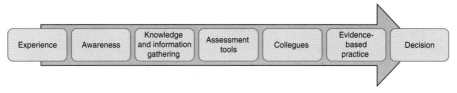

Fig. 8.11 Factors affecting good decision-making. (National Health Service Education for Scotland, 2022.)

RELATIONSHIP BETWEEN SITUATIONAL AWARENESS AND DECISION-MAKING AND THE LINK TO PATIENT SAFETY

There is a clear relationship between situational awareness and decision-making. People who demonstrate a high degree of situational awareness are found to make high quality decisions (Stanners and French, 2005). The decisions made affect the actions, and ultimately the outcomes. Similar to situational awareness, decisions made by individuals will also depend on their competence and skill levels. Decisions can be fast, intuitive, analytical and evidence-based (National Health Service Education for Scotland, 2022). Good decision-making is based on a number of factors that are outlined in Fig. 8.11.

Decisions can be simple or complex. Within healthcare, there can be decisions that require more than one individual or process to make a decision. The Swiss cheese model by Reason (Bajracharya et al., 2019) is based on the understanding that every step in a process, or every layer of a system, has weaknesses that can lead to failure (Fig. 8.12). The systems and processes are like layers of Swiss cheese, the random holes represent the weaknesses at each stage. Active or latent errors can occur as a result of these weaknesses; however, each layer of cheese can also act as a defence against the error. If an individual or team decision leads to an error, then the more this occurs in the system, the greater the risk of an error occurring. This can have a significant impact on the outcome and compromise patient safety.

WHY NURSES AND OTHER HEALTHCARE PROFESSIONALS MAKE THE DECISIONS THEY DO

Nurses and other healthcare professionals make decisions based on their own skills and experiences. Decision-making involves choosing from a variety of alternative courses of action or inaction (National Health Service Education for Scotland, 2022). Nurses and other healthcare professionals may make decisions based on their beliefs or biases about a situation that compel them to take a certain course of action or inaction (Baer, 2017). There are 10 forms of bias that may affect decision-making within healthcare (National Health Service England, 2022):

1. **Affinity bias:** People share the same qualities or affinities with one another.
2. **Attribution bias:** Certain judgements or assumptions are made about attributes.

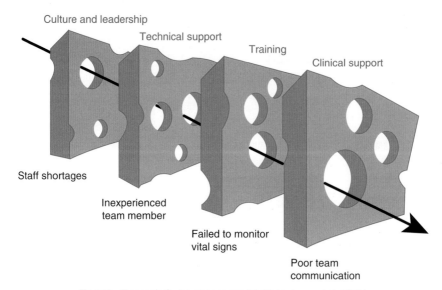

Fig. 8.12   Reason's Swiss cheese model. (Bajracharya et al. 2019.)

3. Beauty bias: Judgements are based on beauty.
4. Conformity bias: People agree with the majority of their group to conform.
5. Confirmation bias: More weight is given to a situation based on personal experiences.
6. Gender bias: Judgements are based on an assumption or a belief about gender.
7. Halo bias: The focus is on one great feature of an individual and a decision is based on this.
8. Contrast effect: A decision is made based on the contrast of an individual in comparison with another.
9. Ageism: Judgements and beliefs based on age.
10. Name bias: Judgements and beliefs are based on the name of a person.

Depending on the situation, these biases may have positive or negative impacts on decision-making. Sometimes these decisions are made unconsciously because people are not aware of their own biases.

Martha Mills was a 15-year-old who tragically died after sustaining a pancreatic injury from the handlebar of her bicycle. She was admitted to the hospital and developed sepsis during her stay. The coroner's report highlighted that Martha's care worsened because of lack of coordination between the paediatric hepatologists and the paediatric intensivists (National Health Service Education for Scotland, 2022). According to Martha's mother, the coroner's report revealed that high status consultants had a dismissive attitude to less senior colleagues, which made them reluctant to do the right thing (Myers & Briggs Foundation, 2022). Her mother stated, 'Martha died because of inflated egos'. Unfortunately, Martha's death is an example of individual bias that may have affected decision-making. The coroner concluded that action should be taken to prevent future deaths.

What Are the Elements of Decision-making?

Good decision-making in healthcare requires a combination of experience and skills (National Health Service Education for Scotland, 2022) including:

- Pattern recognition: Look for cues based on experience that help to inform the decision-making process.
- Critical thinking: The ability to appraise information based on evidence, be aware of any biases and use problem solving skills and creativity.
- Communication skills: Include active listening, knowing the stakeholders, understanding styles of communication and being able to adapt to and adopt styles.
- Evidence-based approaches: Use evidence from what does and does not work well to ensure the correct outcome for an individual, and to know where and how to seek information.
- Teamwork: Approach other members of a multidisciplinary team to ask for help and support, have a clear pathway for escalation and deescalation in the team, listen and be respectful to colleagues and know the roles and responsibilities of other team members.
- Sharing learning: Teach and learn from one another to ensure that everyone has the skills and competencies to fulfil their roles, and gain feedback regarding decisions made formally and informally through peers, mentors and supervisors.

DECISION-MAKING MODELS

Decision-making is dependent on individuals and the choices that they make. There appear to be many variables that can impact how individuals arrive at their decisions. However, the work of the Myers & Briggs Foundation (2022) found that individual behaviour is orderly and consistent due to basic differences in the ways that individuals prefer to use their perception and judgment. They proposed that people have preferences in the way they perceive and make judgement based on four basic principles:

1. How they view the world.
2. How they prefer to interpret information.
3. How they prefer to make decisions.
4. How they deal with the outside world.

Based on these principles people are either:

1. Introvert (I) or Extrovert (E)
2. Sensing (S) or Intuition (N)
3. Thinking (T) or Feeling (F)
4. Judging (J) or Perceiving (P)

There are 16 different personality types based on these principles. For example, an individual may be an Introvert (I), Sensing (S), Feeling (F), Perceiving (P) (i.e. an ISFP) or an Extrovert (E), Intuition (N), Thinking (T), Judging (J) (i.e. an ENJT). Based on the combination of their personality types an individual will typically behave in a certain way. For example, individuals with an ISFP personality type are 'Quiet, friendly, sensitive and kind. Enjoy the present moment, what's going on around them. Like to have their own space and to work within their own time frame. Loyal and committed to their values and to people who are important to them. Dislike disagreements and conflicts, do not force their opinions or values on others' (Myers & Briggs Foundation, 2022).

A person will make a decision based on either thinking or feeling. Thinking personality types are very logical and analytical whereas people who are feeling tend to go with what people care about and the points of view of the people around them.

Being aware of individual personality types can support individuals and teams to understand how they will react in certain situations. This information can also support individuals in knowing their strengths and where they require support. It can also be helpful for designing systems and processes to understand whether a decision will require thinking or feeling.

Nurses integrate analysis and synthesis of intuition alongside analytical objective data when making decisions. When these are integrated, the quality and safety of patient care increases (Johansen and O'Brien, 2016).

The healthcare environment allows for both intuitive and analytical decisions. Intuitive decisions are often quick and can support an individual in making fast paced decisions. For more complex and difficult issues, slower analytical clinical reasoning is beneficial for making decisions (Gasaway, 2021). Nurses make decisions using four strategies—analytical, intuitive, analytical-intuitive and intuitive-analytical—and favour a certain style of decision-making besides considering other variables.

Supporting Good Situational Awareness and Decision-making in Healthcare

This chapter has focused on how poor situational awareness affects the outcomes for individuals, teams and organisations. Mitigation of poor situational awareness and decision-making is pivotal to ensuring safe, effective person-centred care.

Human factors consider how to optimise human performance through better understanding of individual behaviours and interactions with others and their environment. There are many ways to encourage good situational awareness and decision-making in healthcare.

Simulation Training

Simulation training in healthcare can help support people develop their situational awareness, critical thinking and decision-making skills (Patient Safety Network, 2017). It allows opportunity to learn new skills, engage in deliberate practice, receive focused and real-time feedback and bridge the gap between classroom training and real-world clinical experiences (Simulation Matters, 2013). In addition, it provides an opportunity for individuals and teams to work together and understand how they may react in certain situations.

A very simple simulation activity many of us have experienced is an unannounced fire alarm. We are reacting to a potentially hazardous situation and will either have to respond on an individual or team level. The principle being that, should a real fire occur, the practice will support correct decision-making during an actual event and hopefully save lives.

There are various simulation training methods, including specific task training for a particular focus area, such as full scale simulators, virtual reality simulation and actor-based simulation training (Patient Safety Network, 2017).

Objective structured clinical examination (OSCE) is a simulation method predominantly used in healthcare staff assessments. It allows for a structured observation of an individual or team under certain conditions.

Environmental Modifications

Environmental modifications can support effective situational awareness and decision-making when individuals or teams are encouraged to do the right things for people.

Signage may be used to ensure that there are visual cues or warning systems to encourage the staff to do the right things.

Infection prevention and control has been of significance during the COVID-19 pandemic. Many healthcare and other organisations have encouraged staff to wash their hands (World Health Organization, 2022) as this is the first line of defence in any infection prevention and control measure. Fig. 8.13 presents examples of how organisations encourage staff to make good decisions.

Your 5 moments for hand hygiene

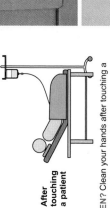

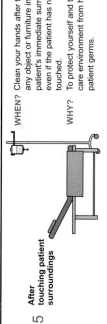

1 Before touching a patient

WHEN? Clean your hands before touching a patient when approaching him/her.

WHY? To protect the patient against harmful germs carried on your hands.

2 Before CLEAN/ASEPTIC procedure

WHEN? Clean your hands immediately before performing a clean/aseptic procedure.

WHY? To protect the patient against harmful germs, including the patient's own, from entering his/her body.

3 After body fluid exposure risk

WHEN? Clean your hands immediately after an exposure risk to body fluids (and after glove removal).

WHY? To protect yourself and the health-care environment from harmful patient germs.

4 After touching a patient

WHEN? Clean your hands after touching a patient and her/his immediate surroundings, when leaving the patient's side.

WHY? To protect yourself and the health care environment from harmful patient germs.

5 After touching patient surroundings

WHEN? Clean your hands after touching any object or furniture in the patient's immediate surroundings—even if the patient has not been touched.

WHY? To protect yourself and the health-care environment from harmful patient germs.

Fig. 8.13 Example of signage.

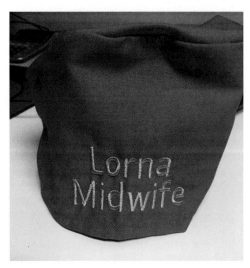

Fig. 8.14 Named surgical hat.

Numerous initiatives are recommended and have been used in healthcare to aid communication within teams to support situational awareness and decision-making.

The Health and Safety Executive highlights using the technique SLAM (stop, look, assess and manage) the task (Edbrookes-Childs et al., 2018). SLAM the task is recommended at the beginning of any new work project, when the work environment has changed and when working with new or different workmates.

Checklists have been introduced to ensure that the right care is provided at the right time and that all aspects of patient care are completed. The sepsis six (Robson and Daniel, 2008) checklist contains six simple things that should be completed within the first hour for an individual suspected to have sepsis. Checklists can communicate actions and outcomes for people (Sepsis Research, 2021).

Safety huddles encourage a focused group of staff to come together to discuss patient care. They improve teamwork and safety because staff can regularly discuss issues in a small group where they are encouraged to contribute and try to mitigate patient risks, which also provides opportunities for reflection and feedback.

To improve communication during caesarean section surgery, the multidisciplinary team wear named surgical hats and scrubs. This allows better communication because everyone can know what disciplines of staff are in the theatre and they are clear about who they are talking to. Fig. 8.14 shows an example of the surgical hat for Lorna, a midwife.

To prevent errors during medication dispensing, a do not disturb at medication administration tabard is worn by nursing staff (Fig. 8.15). This alleviates the interruptions that often cause serious errors.

Significant adverse event reviews (SAER) and local management team reviews are opportunities to improve situational awareness and decision-making. Adverse events are reviewed by a local review team. They are a key source of intelligence about how safe care has been in the past and they have clarity in understanding and improving safety (Healthcare Improvement Scotland, 2019).

Human Factors Education

Developing and embedding human factors knowledge with healthcare staff is key to ensuring safer healthcare (Royal College of Nursing, 2022). If individuals and teams have a better understanding

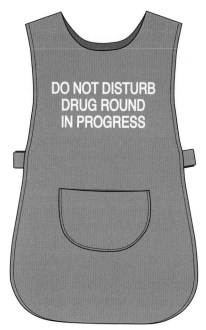

Fig. 8.15 Medication tabard.

of human factors impact on patient outcomes, they are more likely to consider modifications of systems and processes which would enable safer staffing and patient care.

Situation awareness for everyone (SAFE) (Leadership and Worker Involvement Toolkit, n.d.) is an example of a human factors education and improvement programme that targets situational awareness in clinical teams to detect potential deterioration and other risks to children in hospital wards.

In addition to formal human factors education, there are many examples of campaigns that focus on improving patient safety through informing healthcare staff of situational awareness and decision-making.

'Sock it to sepsis' (Sepsis Research, 2021) is a campaign run by Sepsis Research with the aim of increasing awareness of sepsis, how to recognise the signs and symptoms and knowing if the condition of someone with sepsis is deteriorating.

Meningitis Now (2022) has a campaign, 'adults get it too', to help to raise awareness that adults can also get meningitis.

During these campaign periods, staff awareness-raising sessions take place. There are also opportunities to review the identification systems and processes for sepsis or meningitis and simulation training.

Conclusion

Situational awareness and decision-making are critical components of healthcare and directly impact patient safety. In worst-case scenarios, poor situational awareness and decision-making can lead to death or serious harm. It is important to apply a human factors approach to mitigate risks for individuals and teams. Nursing and other healthcare staff should have knowledge and understanding of situational awareness and its impact on decision-making. Simulation training, environmental modifications and human factors education all help to raise awareness and support staff in providing high quality, people-centred care.

References

Ahmed, M., Arora, S., McKay, J., Long, S., Vincent, C., Kelly, M., et al., 2014. Patient safety skills in primary care: a national survey of GP educators. BMC Fam. Pract. 15, 206.

Babiker, A., El Husseini, M., Al Nemri, A., Al Frayh, A., Al Juryyan, N., Faki, M.O., et al., 2014. Health care professional development: working as a team to improve patient care Sudan. J. Paediatr. 14 (2), 9–16.

Baer, M.B., 2017. Your biases and beliefs are impacting your decision-making. Psychol. Today. https://www.psychologytoday.com/ca/blog/empathy-and-relationships/201706/your-biases-and-beliefs-are-impacting-your-decision-making.

Bajracharya, D.C., Karki, K., Lama, C.Y., Joshi, R.D., Rai, S.M., Jayaram, S., et al., 2019. Summary of the international patient safety conference, June 28–29, 2019, Kathmandu, Nepal. Patient Saf. Surg. 13, 36.

BBC News, 2020. Coronavirus: Lockdown Delay 'Cost a Lot of Lives', Says Science Adviser. BBC News, 7 June 2020. https://www.bbc.co.uk/news/uk-politics-52955034.

Benner, P., 2001. From Novice to Expert: Excellence and Power in Clinical Nursing Practice, commemorative ed. Prentice Hall Health, Upper Saddle River.

Berkeley Institute for Data Science, 2022. Situational Awareness Project Description. https://bids.berkeley.edu/research/situational-awareness-dashboard-primary-care-clinicians.

Besnard, D., Greathead, D., Baxter, G.D., 2004. When mental models go wrong. Int. J. Hum. Comput. 60, 117–128.

Brabban, A., Turkington, D., 2002. The search for meaning: detecting congruence between life events, underlying schema and psychotic symptoms. In: Morrison, A.P. (Ed.), A Casebook of Cognitive Therapy for Psychosis. Brunner, Hove, pp. 59–75.

Brennan, P.A., Holden, C., Shaw, G., Morris, S., Oeppen, R.S., 2020. Leading article: what can be done to improve individual and team situational awareness to benefit patient safety? Br. J. Oral Maxillofac. Surg. 58 (4), 404–408.

Bromiley, M., 2011. Clinical human factors group: our history. https://chfg.org/chfg-history/.

Cambridge Dictionary, 2021. Cambridge University Press, Cambridge. https://dictionary.cambridge.org/us/dictionary/english/

Chavin, C., Clostermann, J.P., Hoc, J.M., 2008. Situation awareness and the decision making process in a dynamic avoiding collisions at sea. J. Cogn. Eng. Decis. Mak. 2 (1), 1–23.

Chu, R.Z., 2016. Simple steps to reduce medication errors. Nursing 46 (8), 63–65.

Civil Aviation Authority, 2014. Flight-crew Human Factors Handbook. Civil Aviation Authority, West Sussex.

Clinical Human Factors Group, 2015. Human Factors in Healthcare: Common Terms. chfg-human-factors-common-terms.pdf (websitehome.co.uk).

Davis, N., 2016. A Guide to Situational Awareness. Independent Nurse. https://www.independentnurse.co.uk/content/professional/a-guide-to-situational-awareness/.

Didau, D., 2017. A Novice to Expert Model of Learning. https://learningspy.co.uk/learning/novice-expert-model-learning/.

Dirik, H.F., Samur, M., Interpeler, S.S., Hweison, A., 2019. Nurses identification of medication errors. J. Clin. Nurs. 28 (5–6), 931–938.

Downey, E.L., Andress, K., Schultz, C.H., 2013. External factors impacting hospital evacuations caused by Hurricane Rita: the role of situational awareness. Prehosp. Disaster Med. 28 (3), 264–271.

Drew, T., Võ, M.L., Wolfe, J.M., 2013. The invisible gorilla strikes again: sustained inattentional blindness in expert observers. Psychol. Sci. 24 (9), 1848–1853.

Edbrookes-Childs, J., Hayes, J., Sharples, E., Gondek, D., Stapley, E., Sevdalis, N., et al., 2018. Development of the Huddle Observation Tool for structured case management discussions to improve situation awareness on inpatient clinical wards. BMJ Qual. Saf. 27 (5), 365–372.

Endsley, M.R., 2015. Situation awareness misconceptions and misunderstandings. J. Cogn. Eng. Decis. 9 (1), 4–32.

Endsley, M., 2016. Situational Awareness in Health Care. I-PrACTISE Convention, April 24, 2016, Madison, WI. https://www.youtube.com/watch?v=bBDApnMnf3s.

Endsley, M.R., Jones, D.G., 1996. Casual factors related to errors in situational awareness. In: Endsley, M., Robertson, M. (Eds.), Training for Situational Awareness: Situation Awareness Analysis and Measurement. Laurence Erlbaum Associates, New Jersey.

Fischer, M.A., Kennedy, K.M., Durning, S., Schijven, M.P., Ker, J., O'Connor, P., et al., 2017. Situational awareness within objective structured clinical examination stations in undergraduate medical training - a literature search. BMC Med. Educ. 17 (1), 262.

Fore, A.M., Sculli, G.L., 2013. A concept analysis of situational awareness in nursing. J. Adv. Nurs. 69 (12), 2613–2621.

Gasaway, R., 2021. Using the Simulation Environment to Improve Situational Awareness. Situational Awareness Matters. https://www.samatters.com/using-simulation-environment-to-improve-situational-awareness/.

Gillespie, B.M., Gwinner, K., Fairweather, N., Chaboyer, W., 2013. Building shared situational awareness in surgery through distributed dialog. J. Multidiscip. Healthc. 6, 109–118.

Gilson., R.D., 1995. Special issue preface. Hum. Factors 37 (1), 3–4.

Gleitman, H., Gross, J.J., Reisberg, D., 2010. Psychology, eighth ed. W.W. Norton & Company, New York.

Gonzalez, C., Wimisberg, J., 2007. Situation awareness in dynamic decision making: effects of practice and working memory. J. Cogn. Eng. Decis. Mak. 1 (1), 56–74.

Green, B., Parry, D., Oeppen, R.S., Plint, S., Dale, T., Brennan, P.A., 2017. Situational awareness - what is means for clinicians, its recognition and importance in patient safety. Oral Dis. 23 (6), 721–725.

Gugliotta, A., Vensislavova, P., Garcia-Fernandez, P., Peña-Suárez, E., Eisman, E., Crundall, D., et al., 2017. Are situation awareness and decision making totally conscious processes? Results of a hazard prediction task. Transp. Res. F: Traffic Psychol. 44, 168–179.

Health and Safety Executive, 1999. Reducing Error and Influencing Behaviour. https://www.hse.gov.uk/pubns/books/hsg48.htm.

Healthcare Improvement Scotland, 2019. Learning from Adverse Events through Reporting and Review: A National Framework for Scotland. Healthcare Improvement Scotland, Edinburgh.

Healthcare Safety Investigation Branch, 2022. Weight-based Medication Errors in Children. https://hsib-kqcco125-media.s3.amazonaws.com/assets/documents/final-report-weight-based_medication-errors-in-children.pdf.

Hinshaw, K., 2016. Human factors in obstetrics and gynaecology. Obstet. Gynaecol. Reprod. Med. 26 (12), 368–370.

InnerDrive, 2022. 4 Ways to Overcome Cognitive Overload in Your Students. https://blog.innerdrive.co.uk/4-ways-to-overcome-cognitive-overload.

Integrated Human Factors, 2022. 5 Aviation Accidents Caused by Human Factors. https://www.ihfapac.com/5-aviation-accidents-caused-by-hf-2/.

Johansen, M.L., O'Brien, J.L., 2016. Decision making in nursing practice: a concept analysis. Nurs. Forum 51 (1), 40–48.

Kentish-Barnes, N., Morin, N., Cohen-Solal, Z., Cariou, A., Demoule, A., Azoulay, A., 2021. The lived experience of ICU clinicians during the coronavirus disease 2019 outbreak: a qualitative study. Crit. Care Med. 49 (6), e585–e597.

Lamming, L., Montague, J., Crosswaite, K., Faisal, M., McDonach, E., Mohammed, M.A., et al., 2021. Fidelity and the impact of patient safety huddles on teamwork and safety culture: an evaluation of the Huddle up for Safer Healthcare (HUSH) project. BMC Health Serv. Res. 21 (1), 1038.

Leadership and Worker Involvement Toolkit, n.d. Knowing What Is Going on Around You (Situational Awareness). https://assets.grenfelltowerinquiry.org.uk/ (Accessed 14.02.24).

Liao, Q., Cowling, B., Lam, W.T., Ng, M.N., Fielding, R., 2010. Situational awareness and health protective responses to pandemic influenza A (H1N1) in Hong Kong: a cross sectional study. PLoS One 5 (10), e13350.

Lowe, D.J., Ireland, A.J., Ross, A., Ker, J., 2016. Exploring situational awareness in emergency medicine: developing a shared mental model to enhance training and assessment. Postgrad. Med. J. 92 (1093), 653–658.

Marcus, L.J., McNulty, E.J., Flynn, L.B., Henderson, J.M., Neffenger, P.V., Serino, R., et al., 2020. The POP-DOC Loop: a continuous process for situational awareness and situational action. Ind. Mark. Manag. 88, 272–277.

Maslow, A.H., 1943. A theory of human motivation. Psychol. Rev. 50 (4), 370–396.

Maslow, A.H., 1954. Motivation and Personality. Harper & Row Publishers, New York.

Mcdreeamie-musings, 2019. The Good the Bad and the (Can Be) Ugly: The Three Parts of Cognitive Overload. https://mcdreeamiemusings.com/blog/2019/10/15/the-good-the-bad-and-the-can-be-ugly-the-three-parts-of-cognitive-load.

McIntosh, C., 2018. Situational Awareness and Decision Making – More than Technology. https://www.link edin.com/pulse/situational-awareness-decision-making-more-than-chris-mcintosh.

Meningitis Now, 2022. Adults Get it Too. https://www.meningitisnow.org/support-us/news-centre/public-affairs/campaigns/current-campaigns/#adults-get-it-too.

Murphy, J.G., Dunn, W.F., 2010. Medical errors and poor communication. Chest 138 (6), 1292–1293.

Myers & Briggs Foundation, 2022. MBTI Basics. https://www.myersbriggs.org/my-mbti-personality-type/mbti-basics/.

National Health Service Education for Scotland, 2022. What Is Clinical Decision Making? https://www.eff ectivepractitioner.nes.scot.nhs.uk/clinical-practice/what-is-clinical-decision-making.aspx#:~:text=Clinical %20decision%20making%20is%20a,Good%20decisions%20%3D%20safe%20care.

National Health Service Education for Scotland, 2022. Core Skills of Decision Making. https://www.effectiv epractitioner.nes.scot.nhs.uk/clinical-practice/core-skills-of-decision-making.aspx.

National Health Service England, 2022. Understanding Different Types of Bias. https://nshcs.hee.nhs.uk/abo ut/equality-diversity-and-inclusion/conscious-inclusion/understanding-different-types-of-bias/.

Nursing Theory, 2020. From Novice to Expert. https://nursing-theory.org/theories-and-models/from-novice-to-expert.php (accessed 19.01.2024).

Patient Safety Network, 2017. Simulation Training. https://psnet.ahrq.gov/.

Pollack, A.H., Mishra, S.R., Apodaca, C., Khelifi, M., Haldar, S., Pratt, W., 2020. Different roles with different goals: designing to support shared situational awareness between patients and clinicians in the hospital. J. Am. Med. Inform. Assoc. 28 (2), 222–231.

Psychology Today, 2022. Working memory https://www.psychologytoday.com/intl/basics/memory/work ing-memory.

Public Health England, 2021. COVID-19 Situational Awareness. https://assets.publishing.service.gov.uk/government/uploads/system/uploads/attachment_data/file/1049182/S1356_PHE_Situational_Awareness _Summary_.pdf.

Qazi, A., Qazi, J., Naseer, K., Zeeshan, M., Hardaker, G., Maitama, J.Z., et al., 2020. Analyzing situational awareness through public opinion to predict adoption of social distancing amid pandemic COVID-19. J. Med. Virol. 92 (7), 849–855.

Reader, T.W., Flin, R., Davis, N., 2016. A Guide to Situational Awareness. Independent Nurse Magazine. htt ps://www.independentnurse.co.uk/content/professional/a-guide-to-situational-awareness/.

Robson, W.P., Daniel, R., 2008. The sepsis six: helping people to survive sepsis. Br. J. Nurs. 17 (1), 16–21.

Royal College of Nursing, 2022. Patient Safety and Human Factors. https://rcnlearn.rcn.org.uk/Search/Pati ent-safety-and-human-factors.

SA Technologies, 2021. https://satechnologies.com/about/.

Schulz, C.M., Krautheim, V., Hackemann, A., Kreuzer, M., Kochs, E.F., Wagner, K.J., 2016. Situation aware-ness errors in anesthesia and critical care in 200 cases of a critical incident reporting system. BMC Anaes-thesiol 16, 4.

Sepsis Research, 2021. Sock it to Sepsis. https://sepsisresearch.org.uk/sepsis-awareness/.

She, M., Li, Z., 2017. Team situation awareness: a review of definitions and conceptual models. Conference paper engineering psychology and cognitive ergonomics: performance, emotion and situation awareness. In: Proceedings, Part I, of the 14th International Conference, EPCE 2017, Held as Part of HCI International, vols. 9–14. Vancouver, British Columbia, Canada, pp. 406–415.

Simons, D.J., 2012. Basketball gorilla Trick. https://m.youtube.com/watch?v=vJG698U2Mvo.

Simons, D.J., Chabris, C.F., 1999. Gorillas in our midst. Perception 28 (9), 1059–1074.

Simulation Matters, 2013. Using the Simulation Environment to Improve Situational Awareness - Situational Awareness Matters!. https://www.samatters.com/.

Singh, H., Giardina, T.D., Petersen, L.A., Smith, M.W., Paul, L.W., Dismukes, K., et al., 2012. Exploring situational awareness in diagnostic errors in primary care. BMJ Qual. Saf. 21 (1), 30–38.

Sitterding, M.C., Ebright, P., Broome, M., Patterson, E.S., Wuchner, S., 2014. Situation awareness and inter-ruption handling during medication administration. West. J. Nurs. Res. 36 (7), 891–916.

Stanners, M., French, H.T., 2005. An Empirical Study of the Relationship between Situation Awareness and Decision Making. Australian Government Department of Defence, Defence Science and Technology Organisation Systems Sciences Laboratory, Edinburgh, South Australia.

Stanton, N.A., Chambers, P.R.G., Piggott, J., 2001. Situational awareness and safety. Saf. Sci. 39 (3), 189–204.

Suhonen, R., Scott, P.A., 2018. Missed care: a need for careful ethical discussion. Nurs. Ethics 25 (5), 549–551.

Sweller, J., 1988. Cognitive load during problem solving: effects on learning. Cogn. Sci. 12, 257–285.

The Human Memory, 2022. Short-term (Working) Memory. https://human-memory.net/short-term-working-memory/.

Tower, M., Watson, B., Bourke, A., Tyers, E., Tin, A., 2019. Situation awareness and the decision making process of final-year nursing students. J. Clin. Nurs. 28 (21–22), 3923–3934.

UK Parliament House of Commons Transport Committee, 2021. Factors that increase young and novice crash risk. In: Road Safety Young and Novice Drivers. https://committees.parliament.uk/publications/4871/documents/49009/default/.

UNISON, 2015. Red Alert Unsafe Staffing Levels Rising. UNISON London. https://silo.tips/download/unison-s-staffing-levels-survey-2015-red-alert-unsafe-staffing-levels-rising.

van Merriënboer, J.J., Sweller, J., 2010. Cognitive load theory in health professional education: design principles and strategies. Med. Educ. 44 (1), 85–93.

Way, L.W., Stewart, L., Gantert, W., Liu, K., Lee, C.M., Whang, K., et al., 2003. Causes and prevention of laparoscopic bile duct injuries: analysis of 252 cases from a human factors and cognitive psychology perspective. Ann. Surg. 237 (4), 460–469.

World Health Organization, 2022. The Evidence for Clean Hands. https://www.who.int/teams/integrated-health-services/infection-prevention-control/hand-hygiene.

Young, M.S., Brookhuis, K.A., Wickens, C.D., Hancock, P.A., 2015. State of science: mental workload in ergonomics. Ergonomics 58 (1), 1–17.

Bibliography

Anderson, M., 2021. Situation awareness: making sense of the world. Hum. Factors 101https://humanfactors101.com/topics/situation-awareness/.

Ansari, S.P., Rayfield, M.E., Wallis, V.A., Jardine, J.E., Morris, E.P., Prosser-Snelling, E., 2020. A safety evaluation of the impact of maternity-orientated human factors training on safety culture in a tertiary maternity unit. J. Patient Saf. 16 (4), e359–e366.

Clinical Human Factors Group, 2020. Key Human Factors Messages when Working under Pressure. https://chfg.org/key-human-factors-messages-to-support-the-nhs/.

Curran, E.T., 2015. Outbreak Column 16: cognitive errors in outbreak decision making. J. Infect. Prev. 16 (1), 32–38.

Forte, D.N., Kawai, F., Cohen, C., 2018. A bioethical framework to guide the decision-making process in the care of seriously ill patients. BMC Med. Ethics 19 (1), 78.

Pelegrin, C., 2010. Situation awareness and decision making. Safety First 10, 1–4.

Simons, D.J., Chabris, C.F., 1999. Gorillas in our midst. Perception 28 (9), 1059–1074.

Society of Petroleum Engineers, 2015. Decision Making: What Makes Decision Making Good? https://webevents.spe.org/products/decision-making-what-makes-a-decision-good.

Stubbings, L., Chaboyer, W., McMurray, A., 2012. Nurses' use of situation awareness in decision-making: an integrative review. J. Adv. Nurs. 68 (7), 1443–1453.

Toner, E.S., 2009. Creating Situational Awareness: A Systems Approach. White Paper, Workshop on Medical Surge Capacity, Institute of Medicine Forum on Medical and Public Health for Catastrophic Events, Washington, D.C., 10–11 June 2009.

Wilson, J.R., 2014. Fundamentals of systems ergonomics/human factors. Appl. Ergon. 45 (1), 5–13.

CHAPTER 9

Human Factors from a Leadership Perspective

Mel Newton

1. Discuss recruitment and selection process
2. Describe induction and talent management
3. Describe systems, ethical and compassionate styles of leadership
4. Develop an understanding of power gradients, incivility and psychological safety in relation to teamwork practices
5. Describe the impact of personal effectiveness and the human dimension of change
6. Support the development of reflection and learning

Introduction

This chapter aims to address the key issues of leadership practice, all of which are presented along-side an example which raises questions for consideration. The link between leadership and the relevance of human factors will be further clarified in this chapter. Each section intends to serve as a basis for reflection, and ends with an activity to encourage engagement with the content. This chapter explores the relationship between personal effectiveness as a nontechnical skill and human factors. To identify some of the key themes, a fictitious narrative approach will be employed. Although the scenarios described do not relate to any real events, they are realistic and reflective of contemporary clinical practices. The narrative will comprise evolving professional diary entries of Sarah, who has just taken up the post of a Ward Manager who is responsible for the rehabilitation area for patients who have suffered a stroke. She has a clinical leadership role and her journey throughout the first year at a new hospital gives us an opportunity to understand the key milestones of leadership development.

Recruitment and Selection

DIARY ENTRY 1

Monday 6th September

I am so pleased. I just received my letter of appointment to start my new role at St Mary's Hospital in 4 weeks' time. I have not been to St Mary's, other than for the interview, and so I am excited to see how it operates; the ward looks amazing. I am so scared that I will fail as the manager, just hoping that they will look after me. The letter has me down as Emma, I will have to explain that I am known as Sarah. The joy of having an official first name and being known by another one, typical mother!

The recruitment and selection process for an organisation is the first experience for most staff and the initial opportunity to observe how the organisation operates. The organisational mission statement and vision will likely be evident in the recruitment documentation as well as the values and standards of behaviour expected of all employees. The welcome package may also give practical information, but it will be the people within the organisation that make the impact. For example, Sarah will be able to observe how efficient the process is from her perspective. Is she met and welcomed by someone who is expecting her? Does she have someone to show her the practical aspects of working at St Mary's? Will this 'buddy' become her mentor? Most importantly, will people be friendly and warm towards her? There is an opportunity for negotiating your own terms of employment at the interview stage. Woodward (2005) recounts his missed opportunity to request office and administrative support which would be crucial for his ability to undertake his role as head coach for the England rugby team.

Most recruitment practices have an element of unconscious bias; the selection panel will favour people who look and sound like them (Heffernan, 2019). This is not a deliberate intention; however, the consequences limit and stifle innovations (Syed, 2019). For an organisation to flourish, a diverse workforce is essential and including talent from widely different backgrounds will ensure more creativity and resilience. Therefore as a new leader, Sarah must consider her own personal effectiveness in her position. Personal effectiveness covers those skills and abilities that we need to have, regardless of our job, status or professional background. Personal effectiveness is underpinned by a commitment to reflective practice—to consider what we do, why we do it (must do it) and how we might do it better the next time. It is important that Sarah takes time to reflect upon her own needs and consider what she requires to enable her to become part of the organisation. She should observe how diverse (or not) the people around her appear. Of course, people with different skin colour may share the same kind of life experience and people who look the same may have very different histories; thus, it is important not to make stereotypical judgements. Homogeneity creates a collective blind spot in the organisation. Therefore Sarah should try to keep a 'fresh eyes' perspective and avoid becoming immersed and acclimatised too quickly into the organisational culture. Her personal authenticity and integrity are leadership qualities that are vital to her success. Syed (2019), in his discussion about typical recruitment practices of organisations, distinguishes between rebels and clones, and suggests that most organisations recruit clones which reduces the diversity of ideas. Since Sarah has joined St Mary's after working at a different hospital, she will have a different perspective, and this alone can be invaluable. However, she needs to be encouraged to share her ideas and experiences. Heath and Heath (2013) point out that opportunities are missed when new recruits are not listened to.

From a human factors' perspective, interactions between people and the environment, tasks and processes and structures cannot be overlooked (CIEHF, 2018). People work within complex structures and it may become easy to focus on the human dimension and disregard the influence of other aspects. For example, a good indicator of how processes are implemented is observing what the process for welcoming new staff members to an organisation is and whether feedback from staff is requested to inform and improve the experience for subsequent new members. Consider your own organisation; are new recruits asked to give feedback on their recruitment experience? This is a time-limited opportunity because new staff do not stay new for very long and often want to blend in as quickly as possible.

EXERCISE 9.1

Think about your own experience as a new person in a team or organisation. What made the biggest impact on you? Where you work, are the recruitment processes 'values based' or 'strengths based' and what is the implicit message behind them? What alternative recruitment strategies are there?

As a leader, how do you welcome new members to the team and how much time do you invest? How do you ensure they are well supported to reduce the likelihood of them being involved in a patient safety incident due to unfamiliarity with systems and processes?

Induction

DIARY ENTRY 2

Monday 18th September

I met a lovely lady from human resources today, not sure who she was, but I sat in a small room and watched the corporate videos; apparently that was my induction to St Mary's. I have been teamed up with a buddy from another ward, but she was absent today (sick leave, I think). The ward staff seem nice and busy but friendly. Apparently, I share the office with the team physiotherapy lead who has the desk near the window. He explained that all the policies are on the intranet and once I get my log-in, I will be able to access them. Still not sure who arranges my log-in?

Consider your own organisational inductions. It may have been a while since you experienced being the new person in the team; thus, you might want to think about how you welcome subsequent people into your team. From a leadership perspective, how might Sarah feel about organisation, based upon the human interactions rather than what she reads or learns from watching the corporate video and the formal induction processes? The expression 'culture eats strategy for breakfast' fits well. Can you hazard a guess about what the perceived culture might be? Most definitions about culture refer to 'the way things are done around here'. How would you determine your own team or organisational culture? Do you have access to the results from staff surveys of your organisation? What can you determine from the results and how they are presented to you? There are numerous ways to define culture, but it might be worth exploring the notion of a safety culture defined as 'the combined individual and group values, attitudes, competencies and patterns of behaviour that determine the overall commitment to patient safety' (Bowie, 2010). Safety culture could be an aspirational goal for Sarah to strive towards and she will need a team with potential to succeed.

The National Health Service (NHS) trusts have a talent management strategy used to identify individual and team potential and facilitate individual, team and organisational growth and development (NHS Leadership Academy, 2024a). This could be a function of an organisational development team. Succession planning, one aspect of talent management, and individual development plan use are keys to success. Sarah should expect an initial development meeting with her line manager. In this meeting, the organisation goals as well as the contribution Sarah can make in her role to help the organisation succeed in achieving these goals should be discussed. It is important that Sarah prepares for this meeting and identifies her own needs at this time. Once Sarah's personal objectives are negotiated and agreed upon, her team should be made aware of these goals so that they can then identify their own contributions in line with their roles. The organisation vision should be clear, transparent and aspirational. A safety culture concept for the organisation and ward could be an important aspect.

According to the NHS Leadership Academy (2024a), talent management is the systematic attraction, identification, development, engagement, retention and deployment of individuals who have been identified as having particular value to an organisation, either in view of their 'high potential' for the future or because they are fulfilling critical roles. Succession planning is about making the necessary preparations to have the right people ready to fill key roles when vacancies arise. It eliminates the need to recruit for positions that are difficult to fill, allows recruiting to focus on entry-level positions and prevents organisational knowledge loss. A clear and transparent career path can aid staff retention (Timms, 2016). From the early induction period, Sarah should have an idea about where she sees herself in the near future and, if possible, be able to identify the knowledge and skills she needs to develop to be effective. A starting point might be to consider education and training opportunities, opportunities to shadow senior staff or observe senior executive board meetings to enhance understanding about how the organisation operates and decisions are made. The KPIs for the organisation should be explicitly disclosed during the meeting.

From a human factors' point of view, we can consider how easy (or not) it might be for new staff to undertake their roles. For example, to access patient laboratory results, which is an essential and integral part of patient care, how many steps does the process comprise to access? Consider allocating a staff sign in number and password. Indeed, this is often not a quick and simple process because of compliance with security issues. This requires the coordination of several departments, such as the human resources department, information technology (IT) systems and pathology laboratory department.

EXERCISE 9.2

What are the key performance indicators (KPIs) for your organisation? How easy is it to locate the KPIs? Are they reflected in your professional development plan?

Try to see how your organisation responds to the National Talent Management Strategy. Are there opportunities for leaders to undertake further training events?

Do you have access to your Regional Leadership Academy and are the resources available? In addition to leadership courses, will there be other training events such as coaching courses, resilience courses and other professional development events for anyone working in the NHS? You might want to subscribe to the organisation e-newsletter for details.

Power Gradient

DIARY ENTRY 3

Monday 2nd October

Oh my word! What have I taken on! The consultant is a scary person. She expects me to lead the ward round and introduce her to each patient by giving her a summary of the care and treatment. I am completely out of my comfort zone; we did not work like this before. I spend nearly a full day preparing for the ward round. The senior staff nurse has just gone onto maternity leave, so I feel completely lost.

The potentially intimidating relationship between the ward manager and the consultant is a source of concern because it can influence other team members and result in substandard care which compromises patient safety. The ability to manage the expectations that other people have of us can be challenging. For example, Sarah needs to consider how to be courageous and initiate a conversation with the consultant to discuss the expectations of Sarah and her role. The timing of the meeting will be crucial to its success and she may decide to wait until she has a clearer understanding of their relationship. This is a difficult proposition; however, it is the most effective way to deal with the situation. When planning the conversation, it is important to consider the timing, venue and content of the conversation—if possible, it should be held in a private area during a time when both participants do not feel rushed and are not needed elsewhere. A coffee break, to make the conversation less formal, might be worth considering. An honest and equal exchange of thoughts and ideas about the best way to manage the professional relationship would be ideal and include opportunities for both to negotiate and compromise. While this may seem daunting for Sarah, it is essential that she is able to assert herself and explain her role and how she will fulfil it. Only through exploration of assumptions held by both people will they be able to find a middle ground. There is no doubt that Sarah will need to draw upon excellent interpersonal communication skills.

If you have not seen the video *Just a Routine Operation* (https://www.youtube.com/watch?v=J zlvgtPIof4) about the care of Elaine Bromiley, take time to watch it; or if you have seen it, maybe watch it again. As you watch, please pay attention to the way the nurses interact with the medical consultants, especially when a bed in the intensive therapy unit (ITU) is arranged. Try to make observations about the leadership (or lack of), decision-making, team working and communication styles. In additional, it is worthwhile reading the 'Independent report on the death of Elaine Bromiley' (Bromiley, n.d.). In that report, the significance of embedding a human factors approach and a learning culture is reiterated. Donaldson (2002) reports the need for organisations to learn from past significant events so that lessons can be learned.

It is important for Sarah to remember that she is in a leadership position with some authoritative power and others will respond to her role in the organisation. She needs to be careful about using her positional power effectively and recognise it for what it is, including its benefits and limitations. For example, she will be expected to exert authority with care and compassion, although there may be occasions where she feels 'gagged' and unable or unwilling to voice concerns that could be perceived as provocative or noncorporate. Personal tensions may arise if she is expected to advocate for something that she has no real confidence about. Consider the leadership dilemma; how could she resolve these tensions? What support mechanisms might she try to employ?—for example, support from peers and managers, clinical supervision, coaching, and mentoring.

Heffernan (2019) discusses the thorny issue which she calls 'wilful blindness', wherein individuals and organisations do not see what is often obvious. She recounts experiences of major organisations that failed to listen when employees tried to share concerns, and refers to 'Cassandras' from mythology who can see potential pitfalls but which are ignored or ridiculed. Often leaders live in 'echo chambers' where they are only exposed to voices that share their perspective. Effective leaders need to actively seek out dissonant voices and the naysayers so that they can guard against becoming wilfully blind to potential disasters and encourage staff to develop a safety voice. Syed (2019) refers to dissonant voices and a constructive dissent. He talks about a 'steep authority gradient' wherein questioning a senior person could be perceived as a threat to status. He recounts an example from the 1970s—an airplane accident that resulted when an engineer did not voice concerns about a pilot's decision, due to hierarchal deference norms. This is in contrast to Weick and Sutcliffe (2015) who refer to 'deference to expertise' as one of the five principles of highly reliable organisations. They offer examples from fire and rescue services—a chief fire officer will adopt and maintain a mindset of uncertainty so that his rank and status do not become confused for expertise in a situation new to him.

EXERCISE 9.3

In terms of Sarah looking after her emotional well-being, what actions can she take? How can Sarah start to get feedback about how others and her staff see her?

How do others see you? You might want to read more about emotional intelligence; there are good resources available on YouTube and Ted Talks (e.g. Brene Brown 'Call to Courage' https://www.youtube.com/watch?v=rfxKj8GVVxU).

Weick and Sutcliffe (2015) suggest that simple questions can help identify if or how deference to expertise is practiced.

- Do people respect the nature of one another's work?
- Is expertise and experience valued above hierarchical rank?
- When something unusual happens, can people identify who would have the expertise to help?
- How easy is it to get expert help when something happens and people do not know how to respond?
- When something unexpected happens, do the most highly qualified people help with sensemaking and decision-making, regardless of rank?

Compassionate Care and Compassionate Leadership

DIARY ENTRY 4

Monday 7th October

Today I had my initial performance review (IPR) with Sally, she is the matron for the directorate. She was so lovely; we had a cup of coffee and it seemed like a chat rather than IPR. She was keen to get to know me and asked about my previous experiences. She has some great ideas about my professional development and is asking me to think about obtaining a leadership master's degree.

She explained that the ward had some issues, and that the consultant was well known for being rude and frosty. She said that together we could pull the ward around and make it excellent. The hospital is just about to launch an 'Incivility Costs Lives' campaign which sounds interesting. Sally talked about compassionate leadership which also sounds interesting.

Compassionate care and compassionate leadership go hand in hand. Trzeciak and Mazzarelli (2019) coined the expression 'compassionomics' and write about compassionate healthcare in the United States of America. In their book, they demonstrate that compassion can be scientifically identified and analysed. They provide a rigorous review of the human connections between medical staff and patients, and how impactful feeling cared about can be in terms of both healthcare and finance. Although the content is patient focused, the reality is that all people (staff as well as patients) thrive and flourish in caring environments.

Regarding compassionate leadership, the works of Michael West (2021) and Brene Brown (2018) are good starting points. West, as part of The King's Fund (West et al., 2014), explored the concept of commitment leadership. In the publication, The King's Fund looked at how teams can best work together. The move away from transformational/transactional leadership (Burns, 1978) suggests that a devolved style of leadership could be the most effective—incorporating shared leadership in the team to achieve success by using the talents and skills from the team. In the transformational/transactional leadership style, the leader is the main point of attention and holds the power. This is a stark contrast to the servant leadership approach, in which the aim of the leader is to facilitate team development. In this approach, the leader 'leads from behind' and assists the team to maximise potential (Spears, 2010). Ten qualities are identified in servant leadership:

- Listening
- Empathy
- Healing
- General awareness
- Persuasion
- Conceptualisation
- Foresight
- Stewardship
- Commitment to the growth of people
- Building community

More recently, West (2020) discussed the importance of people freeing themselves from the constraints of job titles so that they can work towards blurring organisational boundaries. He refers to 'softening of hierarchies', indicating that the rank or status of a person is less important than the contribution they can make during a crisis situation, such as the coronavirus disease 2019 (COVID-19) pandemic. He goes on to say that compassion is a core value in healthcare and echoes the findings of Trzeciak and Mazzarelli (2019), with examples of how compassionate preoperative care by an anaesthetist can reduce the postoperative requirement for opiates for the patient by 50% with a shortened in hospital stay. The need for leaders to demonstrate compassion is equally important. West (2020) suggests that leaders should take time and effort to truly understand the challenges that other people face and that by 'listening with fascination' leaders can empathise with others. He recommends that there are four key behaviours that leaders can demonstrate. Firstly, attending to those we lead, meaning that leaders should actively listen and be present when engaging with others. Secondly, leaders should understand the challenges that other people face by initiating conversations and dialogue. Thirdly, leaders can empathise with others and feel what their experiences are like. Finally, leaders can help others by removing obstacles and ensuring that resources which would help develop skills and knowledge are made available.

Brene Brown's 'Call to Courage' is approximately 50 minutes long and is worth watching. In her books, *Dare Greatly* (2013) and *Dare to Lead* (2018), she shares effective messages about the individual need and responsibility to step up to a leadership role. Brown describes herself as a researcher of shame and vulnerability. She writes from a research informed perspective about the courage to show vulnerability and she aims to dismiss the myth that vulnerability is a weakness.

Furthermore, West (2020) emphasises the need for self-compassion and states that it is vital for leaders to pay attention to their own needs and take action to care for themselves. He suggests that leaders must spend quality time with people they love and who love them. These help influence leaders in their work environments to build belonging and trust and develop cultures of organisational compassion.

EXERCISE 9.4

What leadership style would you like to adopt? How do you think others see you? How can you go about getting an accurate picture about your blind spots? You might want to check out Johari's Window (Luft and Ingham, 1955) for an activity.

Can you list different leadership styles?

How would you describe the leadership within your own organisation? How visible are the leaders and why might this be important?

Incivility

DIARY ENTRY 5

Monday 15th October

I am so angry today. Dr. Monster (my new name for her) raised her voice at me in front of everyone. I was flustered and misidentified a patient and gave the incorrect information. She was furious with me, to the point that her face went red!

Incivility is a term used to describe rudeness. Chris Turner's TED Talk addresses the issue of incivility, and several healthcare organisations have adopted a 'Civility Saves Lives' campaign. The potential patient harm that can result from incivility has been documented by Porath (2016) and evidence suggests that it not only affects the person who directly experiences the rude behaviour of another person, but also the witnesses. Incivility is now better understood, and the time effect is better acknowledged. Therefore if a staff member witnesses the rude behaviour of another person, they become less likely to be helpful or willing to respond to requests for assistance. This knock-on effect is significant and the reason incivility really can affect patient safety.

It is important that Sarah knows her own personal and professional values. As Covey (2020) suggests, a leader needs to think and act in a principled way; but to do this, a leader must firstly understand their own principles. An exercise to do this could include reflecting about what is important to you and thinking about a personal creed or mission statement. This activity takes time and, as with emotional work, it can be energy intensive.

Firstly, identify themes that motivate or drive you—for example, money, family, partner, ambition or recognition. You may feel that family is your main concern in life, but if challenged, how would this stand up? For example, if you promised your family to undertake an activity and then you had a pending deadline for some work, what would you do? Would you rather disappoint the family or the manager? The point of this exercise is to identify what your principles are, rather than what they should be. Of course, once identified, you can decide to change them. An authentic, principled leader is more likely to be effective; followers soon recognise when a leader says one thing but demonstrates behaviours that contradict what they say. This is important when thinking about role modelling behaviour for staff. If a leader sends an e-mail at 8 p.m. but says that they believe staff should rest when not on duty, there will be confusion about what is said and what is done. However, if a leader says that they want staff to look after their own well-being and rest when not on duty, the leader must demonstrate that by leaving work on time, taking lunch and recovery breaks and not working excessively when not on duty. This is a tough call for many leaders, but it is vital. Covey (2020) discusses authentic leadership and suggests that leaders start with the end in mind—meaning, they should consider how they want to be remembered. What will your legacy be?

An example of a personal leadership philosophy:

1. I believe a leader should be a positive role model, accessible, approachable and highly visible.
2. I believe a leader should inspire a shared vision and recognise a future related to the mission, vision, core values and key priorities of the organisation.
3. I believe that professional governance will empower staff to challenge policies, procedures and practices to improve the workplace environment and patient care experiences.
4. I believe people perform at their best depending on the tools they have; I will reward, recognise and celebrate contributions of individuals.
5. I believe in psychological safety for patients, visitors and staff so that people feel comfortable and safe reporting unsafe practices.
6. I believe in our mission to guide the actions and decision-making of the team.

7. I believe in a culture of ownership so that people can be creative and innovative.
8. I believe in lifelong learning and taking responsibility for my own growth and development.
9. I believe communication should be open, honest, ethical and transparent.
10. I believe in setting SMART (specific, measurable, attainable, relevant, time-bound) goals to measure progress toward key priorities; results are important.
11. I believe in collaboration to ensure good representation and inclusivity to accomplish shared visions and goals.
12. I believe that a leader is a relationship manager, and a circle of influence is more important than authority or control.

A leadership philosophy can be shared with a team so that they know what to expect from the leader and how the leader is expected to respond to situations (adapted from Dent, 2016).

EXERCISE 9.5

What is your personal mission statement? What principles do you hold dear? You might want to have a professional conversation with other people about their personal mission statements. A team 'values clarification' exercise is worth undertaking to verify that the whole team is committed to the same values. Once values are agreed upon, you have a standard to measure each other against.

Have you reviewed the NHS Constitution lately? How does this compare to your Organisational Mission Statement and how does that compare to your departmental or ward philosophy? Further, how does that compare to your own mission statement? Are there areas of overlap or are there significant differences?

Systems Leadership
DIARY ENTRY 6

Monday 22nd November
I am so excited; the hospital has decided to have a dedicated stroke team comprising all disciplines. We are going to start a task group to coordinate the care for all patients from the moment that they present with a stroke. This includes prehospital care, accident and emergency (A&E), a stroke unit, rehabilitation services, discharge coordination and community services. It is going to be amazing; we will all work together for the benefit of the patient and families.

Systems leadership has been defined as, 'the collaborative leadership of a network of people in different places and at different levels in the system creating a shared endeavour and cooperating to make a significant change' (Goss, 2015). The leadership required has had several names such as 'adaptive leadership', 'emergent leadership' and 'systems leadership'; however, the most important characteristic is that the change is new and has not been attempted before. An example is the Chartered Institute for Ergonomics and Human Factors (CIEHF) rapid response attempts to help during the COVID-19 crisis. A team of ergonomists worked together to provide guidance for new UK manufacturers to make ventilators for patients with COVID-19. Hignett et al., (2021), a think tank group of people from different professional backgrounds, came together with one key purpose and created a synergistic approach in which the overall outcome was more important than any individual contribution.

This is an important concept for a complex healthcare organisation. Heroic leadership traits were once revered; however, this is no longer the case. Effective leaders need to manoeuvre in various working environments and engage with others who may have equal positional power or authority from different organisations.

Each organisation is likely to have a corporate strategy which will state the values and behaviours expected from all staff members. Most strategies will have aspirational statements as targets to stretch the SMART objectives: specific, measurable, attainable, relevant, time-bound.

When you consider the objective for helping a patient in reducing weight, an individual plan is unlikely to be effective on its own. The patient is likely to live with others who influence lifestyle choices, such as partners and children. They may be employed and eat meals at work with colleagues in a social setting. The availability of convenience and takeaway food should be considered as well as the ability to exercise and make healthy food choices. Therefore an individual plan is too simplistic, and a much wider contextual perspective should include social, economic, housing and environmental aspects. This is a system-wide approach. In this approach, leaders from each domain can work together effectively to address their own area of influence so that when combined, they will have a positive overall impact on health at both the population and individual levels.

In developing a dedicated stroke team, Sarah will have to work across organisational and professional boundaries. She has the expertise as the ward manager for the rehabilitative experience, but this is a limited perspective because she does not have the full view of the patient journey. For example, she cannot appreciate the full extent of primary care services and interventions; she will be unaware of the preventative influence of the patient's relationship with their general practitioner (GP) and community nursing team prior to hospital care. The effectiveness of paramedic assessment and services in the accident and emergency department are beyond her as well as the initial acute critical care treatment episode. Therefore the people with the expertise in these areas are equally important to the contribution of a total stroke team. These stakeholders are likely to include primary care staff, paramedic, medical, nursing, pathology laboratory, radiology, physiotherapy, occupational therapy staff as well as nutritional advisors, speech and language therapy staff and numerous others. Therefore Sarah will share her expertise in a systems leadership role whilst recognising that each leader has an equal contribution in ensuring that patients with stroke have the best experience possible.

EXERCISE 9.6

Can you identify where systems leadership might be evident in your working life? Do you work within a multidisciplinary team or an inter-professional team? Do you recognise inter-agency working which would involve working with people outside your own organisation?

See if you can identify your organisational corporate strategy. What leadership style do you observe in your work environment?

Ethical Leadership

DIARY ENTRY 7

Monday 3rd December
Today I saw something that really upset me—one of the health care assistants was abrupt with a patient when he thought no one was around and he was leaving the ward to go home. He is usually good with patients but seems a bit off lately. I need to address this tomorrow first thing. Not sure what approach to take.

Personal effectiveness is a key leadership attribute and personality influences this. It is worth taking time to become self-aware as an initial step; one of the best ways is to try to understand your own personality. There are numerous models and methods for doing this, such as Insights, Myers-Briggs Type Indicator (MBTI) (Lisle Baker, 2004), 360-degree feedback assessments (Hammerley et al., 2014) and the Healthcare Leadership Model (NHS Leadership Academy, 2024b).

When considering ethical behaviour, it is perhaps more appropriate to think about moral responses to situations. The difference between ethics and morality has been discussed by Armstrong (2007) and he makes a case for referring to morality. Moral principles focus on people's conduct, actions and omissions. This is part of the ethics theory addressing 'what should I do?' (Edwards, 2009). Moral principles are ideas and concepts based on fundamental moral values, and can be identified as justice and fairness; examples are moral obligations/duties, such as when you are morally obliged to be a fair leader and to do the fair thing. Moral principles are useful 'action guides' in difficult moral situations such as moral dilemmas. The significance of moral behaviour regarding leadership is relevant because it is the foundation for building a trusting relationship with others. Considering how to respond to difficult and challenging scenarios is a fragile scenario. There can be tension between acting in line with your employment conditions, satisfying your professional responsibilities and staying true to your own moral compass. There are 'worst case scenarios'. Undergoing disciplinary action for failure to follow organisation policy and practices might result in losing your job. Being held accountable to your professional regulation statutory body for failure to comply with the code of conduct could result in losing registration (and subsequently your job and ability to work as a registrant). These scenarios represent a struggle with moral conflict through an inability to demonstrate moral courage when challenged. Considering these three case scenarios, it is most likely staff will compromise on moral behaviour standards.

Sarah needs to be aware of her own personality and natural responses to situations. Although she might feel upset about what she has witnessed, she can attempt to compartmentalise this response and try to reach out and understand potential reasons (not excuses) why the healthcare assistant (HCA) behaved in an unusual and unexpected way with a patient. She could reflect upon her leadership principles to help her adapt a behaviour in line with her values and moral compass. For example, she might consider showing respect for the HCA by recognising that there could be something impacting his ability to uphold the usual high standards of care, such as additional stress in a homelife situation that has not been disclosed. Emotional and cognitive overload can impair individual performance and result in a downward spiral. As a leader, Sarah might be in a position to make a difference, such as considering rotation between day and night duty rostering for stressed and stretched-out staff, giving rest days at shorter intervals and preventing excessively long shift patterns. There may be other ways to support staff by ensuring they rotate tasks equally so that a repetitive work pattern does not become tedious. A creative and collective approach can be taken to engage with staff to resolve potentially stressful work patterns. For example, for a patient at risk of falling, often a member of the care team might be allocated to provide one-on-one individualised care. If the patient has dementia, this could be challenging to manage in a sensitive and compassionate way for long periods of time. Compassion fatigue among care staff can have a detrimental effect on patient and family experiences. By sharing the responsibility across the care team for 1–2 hours at a time, the individual members can provide sensitive care knowing that they will be relieved.

EXERCISE 9.7

What do you understand about the need to be courageous? Have you had tensions at work where your moral compass had to be checked? Are you be able to reflect upon a time where it was difficult to do the 'right thing'?

What do you understand by the expression 'moral injury'?

Have you experienced compassion fatigue, and can you identify how that feels for you?

Appreciative Inquiry
DIARY ENTRY 8

Monday 2nd March
   I need to talk to Sally, the matron. We have a new junior doctor, and I am worried about her. She does not ask any questions and tries to impress the others. Julie, the HCA, said that Dr. Howard could not take blood from a patient but just kept on trying. The poor patient had bruises up and down her arm but did not want to complain.

Appreciative inquiry can be a tool to highlight key learning elements from an incident without apportioning blame. There are topics with keywords that can be used to facilitate a conversation to fully understand what happened in an event:

- The starting point is likely to be a *definition and outline* for the purpose of the meeting. Questions can include, 'What drew us to this inquiry? What is the deeper and desired outcome? Do we have consent for sharing the learning points?'
- In the *discovery part* of the conversation, a participant would be asked to describe what happened in as much detail as possible and prompts may be used. Some key questions in this section might include a reflection upon things that went well or had a positive impact. Attention is given to what was good and the things that were valued about the interaction such as the way people worked together, or safety practices that were observed. The reflection and benefit of hindsight might be discussed to think about what could have been done differently. Suggestions about enhancements and support for improvement could be considered.
- The next aspect for an appreciative inquiry could be *dream* consideration. The respondent is asked to list three wishes to improve the care experience. What would they like to be done differently? How can patient safety be enhanced and what would a perfect scenario look like?
- Then in the *design* section, questions could pertain to what it might take to create a change in this area? How can lessons be learned and disseminated across the organisation? What initial small action steps could be taken and what are the most radical action points? What resources would be needed to meet aspirations and maximise opportunities? What results would be expected? How can we share learning?
- Examples of questions for the *destiny* part of appreciative inquiry could include those concerning challenges that might be encountered and how to overcome them. Who would be included in the action going forward, if support were to be offered?
- Finally, a *summary* of the discussion would include what could be done differently with action points, timeframes and people responsible.

Sarah will need to address the situation with the HCA and Dr. Howard to better understand why Dr. Howard persisted in trying to obtain a blood sample without asking for help. It is easy to jump to conclusions and make assumptions that may or may not be accurate. She will also want to know why the HCA was unable to say anything to Dr. Howard at the time—thus assuming a patient advocate role. To try to prevent a defensive and hostile discussion, it will take skill to adopt an appreciative inquiry approach.

In trying to understand the situation from different perspectives, Sarah will need to suspend her understanding and ask curious questions that may include interprofessional relationships, for example, between Dr. Howard and the consultant, as well as the HCA and medical staff. The dynamics may be different from what Sarah expects. It is also important that Sarah sets the scene about why she needs to know what happened and potential outcomes for the staff. Transparency and honesty will be vital; thus, if disciplinary action is a possible outcome, the staff need to know that prior to the interview.

EXERCISE 9.8

Have you ever been interviewed about a safety incident? If you have, how did it feel? If you need to question someone about an incident or event, how can you do it with compassion?

How would you ask sensitive questions about relationships between different professional groups without appearing to favour one group to another? How would you start your questions (who, where, what, how, why or when)?

Teamwork Practices

DIARY ENTRY 9

Monday 30th April

I am fed up with the bickering between night staff and day staff. Patients should not be washed and ready for day staff to come onto the ward in the morning, they seem to have lost sight of patient-centred care. I have spoken with Sally and she agrees that something must be done. I am going to get the staff onto a rotational roster!

Much has been written about highly functioning teams and the impact that the chief executive officer (CEO) can have on an organisation. In direct contrast to this notion, Brafman and Beckstrom (2006) outline the merits of a leaderless organisation and suggest that decentralisation can facilitate growth and development in industry. They refer to starfish and spider organisations and make the case that organisations are likely to evolve into starfish style organisations with a decentralised power base. This requires a different leadership skill set than what has been traditionally practiced. Rather than a masculine, heroic style of leadership, a more emotionally intelligent, softer and negotiating style may be the way forward to nurture teamwork practices and celebrate differences.

West (2020) discusses the importance of effective teamwork practices and rates teamworking skills as more valuable in times of crisis (such as the COVID-19 pandemic) than technical skills. He asserts that to be effective, teams require a clear and shared vision with defined objectives. There is a need to eliminate professional boundaries and work without hierarchy. The most effective teams value diversity (which can be demographic or professional) so that the contribution of members knowledge, skill, ability and experience can be harnessed for collective success. He goes on to state that 'effective teamworking is core to high quality care, to innovating and to the mental health of staff' (West, 2020, p. 13).

Sarah will need to think very carefully about how she approaches this situation, and she must be clear about her objectives. For example, if she wants staff to have a better understanding of each other's roles, then is rotating an appropriate response? What might the costs be to an individual staff member who may work set days or nights to have a home/work life balance. Can an alternative response provide a better outcome? For example, what about introducing a twilight shift and an early morning start? This option might be more acceptable to the team and could be put forward as one option for staff to consider and cast a vote. If the problem is discussed in an open staff forum, the team could generate alternative options and engage in ownership of the issue.

EXERCISE 9.9

How would you define your work team dynamics?

Can you identify work issues that might benefit from a whole team discussion to try to resolve problems or enhance care provision? Who are the key people involved in an improvement project?

Psychological Safety

DIARY ENTRY 10

Monday 12th May
   I have been so busy with other things that I missed the safety huddles for the last couple of months. Today, I went to see how things were going and it was weird. Each patient was presented as usual, but what was unusual was that there was no discussion about the care and no suggestions about how to make patients' experiences better. The team leader did all the talking and everyone else just listened and took notes.

Psychological safety can best be described as the ability and willingness for a team to speak out without fear of being humiliated or undermined. That is not to say that by speaking out, the person will not be challenged or criticised; however, in a psychologically safe environment, all staff feel able to constructively challenge each other openly so that they perform in a consistently optimal way. They feel enabled to flag legitimate risks without fear of provoking retaliation. Amy Edmonson is a professor who specialises in researching the phenomenon of psychological safety and has observed healthcare teams and teamworking practices (Edmonson, 1999).

There is a growing body of research regarding the use of voice, which is an important part of making patient care safe. The use of voice can indicate how staff use a safety voice or choose not to speak. In the Francis Report (2013), a recommendation was made to train and appoint speak-up guardians for healthcare organisations who would be available to listen to staff concerns about patient safety. This has also been a feature in subsequent reports to encourage staff to speak up about concerns. Based on their extensive research, Reitz and Higgins (2019) offer practical suggestions about the mechanisms for enabling staff to speak up.

Sarah has identified that staff are not participating in the safety huddle and she needs to investigate why this is happening. The culture or climate of the ward appears to have changed while she had not been attending the huddles. It would be too easy to suggest that the team leader alone was responsible for this; it is a collective responsibility, but the climate will be reflective of the leadership approach that has been taken. Sarah needs to develop a strategy for encouraging the staff to voice their concerns.

It should also be acknowledged that staff can make feelings and thoughts known without the use of voice. For example, a shrug of the shoulders can convey a clear message just as eye-rolling or avoiding eye contact can communicate a feeling. The counterpart of speaking is of course listening.

Reitz and Higgins (2019) offer suggestions about how to speak up and listen with skill:

- Do you, as a team, get a chance to reflect on how you communicate with each other?
- When do you think about what it takes for others to say something about concerns and ideas?
- How do you learn and enhance this over time?
- Who do you go to for honest feedback?
- How do you get to hear challenging and different viewpoints?
- When things seem fine, how would you verify this assumption?
- Is there a way to practice different ways of communicating?
- Are there people who will help you to develop this skill?
- Do you create opportunities to communicate differently, make mistakes, experiment and learn?
- Who gets the recognition in the team and for what reasons?
- What behaviour is encouraged?
- What happens when you make a mistake in speaking up or listening?
- What is the narrative about other people speaking up previously?

Try to observe the behaviour of your team members to see how often alternative views are raised. What is the general response to 'the alternative option?'

Personal Effectiveness and Personality

DIARY ENTRY 11

Monday 14th June
   I cannot believe that I have been on the ward so long now. The directorate leaders are being put through an in-house development course about personal effectiveness. We can have our personality type assessed using MBTI; sounds a bit daunting, but I am up for it.

There are several ways to assess personal effectiveness, such as the use of emotional intelligence assessment tools which ask you to rate how you respond to different situations. Most emotional intelligence development theories start with understanding yourself and having a sound self-awareness (Goleman, 1998). Understanding your own key personality is a good starting point for self-awareness. There are different ways to understand personality and most assessment tools work either on personality traits or innate preferences. The essential part of understanding your own personality is to be able to adapt and flex your responses to situations or trigger events. It also allows you to gain insight into how others might see and respond to you. Rather than use this awareness to justify your behaviour, it is important to realise the need to flex to work more effectively with others. Some personality assessment tools such as MBTI are designed to help people appreciate the preference types of others to foster enhanced communication and teamwork practices as well as leadership development.

Self-knowledge entails weeding out everything you have taken on that does not define you. To uncover the real you underneath, you need to get rid of all the programs, messages, images, beliefs, expectations and energies that do not actually belong to you.

When considering the implementation of a change, there are two main aspects to consider— the tools and techniques which can be the hard or anatomical aspects. Thus, deciding which tools and techniques to use, such as rapid PDSA (plan-do-study-act) cycles, Kotter's change model or even the NHS Change Model, might be relevant. However, when it comes to how you take a team with you, there are interpersonal skills to consider which can be referred to as the physiology of the change initiative.

In any change initiative, there are important factors to consider, and the first is the setting or context of the change, including identifying the direction from where the change originates. For example, is the change linked to a directive external of the organisation (Department of Health) or a directive from within the organisation (a department)? Second, identification of the change agent and the role it has is important. The change could be part of team development with devolved responsibility to a group of people. Alternatively, it may be facilitated by a person outside the team or by a leader such as ward manager with the responsibility to make the change. For the most effective change initiatives, an argument can be made to have someone who knows the team be the leader because they will appreciate the dynamics of the team and the personal history of the team members, which could impact the success of the initiative.

Rogers (1995) identified that team members will respond to a 'top down' change in predictable ways. He presented this in a bell-shaped curve that shows how few people will quickly engage and respond positively to the change, most people will adopt the change once it hits a 'tipping point' and a predictable amount of people will respond to the change with reluctance and may try to avoid the change. This is important for the leader to understand so that a strategy can be developed to maximise energy involved and target a communication plan effectively. For example, communicating to the team and expecting everyone to be positive will leave the leader feeling deflated and possibly exhausted; the leader should anticipate reluctance and possible sabotage from a small minority of people. A deeper analysis will also reveal that the people who resist the change are also more likely to be coming from a perspective of fear and may be 'cognitively overloaded' with emotions from nonwork-related events. Consider the member of staff who is going through a divorce or has recently lost a parent and is grieving and then has a work change to deal with.

From a human factors' point of view, we know that systems and processes can either facilitate or hinder work; thus, when an opportunity to change a work pattern emerges, it is vital to try to see it from as many perspectives as possible to ensure the staff have a share and some ownership of the change. This personal investment cannot be overstated.

EXERCISE 9.11

If you had to implement a change at work, such as a seven-day working pattern or a change to the shift pattern, how do you think your team would respond? Can you identify people who would embrace the change and those who would be hesitant (for different reasons)?

Read 'Who Moved My Cheese' by Spencer, and check out at the activities suggested at the end of the book.

Reflection and Learning

DIARY ENTRY 12

Monday 26th August
Well, I can hardly believe that I have been at St Mary's for nearly a whole year. It has had its ups and downs and I have learned so much about myself and the leadership role.

West (2020) advocates for taking time out as a leader to reflect and learn from experience. He suggests that it is essential for individuals, teams and organisations to make space and time to pause and be still. This enables them to take a breath which is essential for well-being and mental health and ensures they are more effective. He recognises that the best teams stop to debrief, undertake an action review or share in a huddle, and are on average 35% to 40% more effective than teams that remain busy at all costs. Cultures of reflection and learning are known to be more innovative.

The Healthcare Leadership Model identifies nine dimensions of leadership behaviour which can be used as a framework to self-assess or can be used as part of a 360-feedback assessment wherein the raters (including self, peers, direct reports and line managers) rate the observed behaviour and offer feedback to the candidate. The dimensions are:

- Inspiring shared purpose
- Leading with care
- Evaluating information
- Connecting service
- Sharing the vision
- Engaging the team
- Holding accountable
- Developing capability
- Influencing for results

For each dimension, raters indicate whether they observe the candidate as demonstrating exemplary, strong, proficient or essential behaviour in the anonymous questionnaire. The results are used by a trained facilitator to provide feedback to the candidate with the intention of helping to set an action plan to enhance leadership behaviour.

EXERCISE 9.12

Consider your own behaviour against the nine dimensions of leadership behaviour.

Conclusion

Due to the increasing demand in healthcare, staff leadership and how we develop as leaders is paramount. This chapter explored many of the components of leadership development, with a focus on reflective practice and how different experiences can support staff to further develop skills required to be effective leaders. Each reflection has a message based on leadership attributes and an activity asking healthcare practitioners to consider themselves in similar situations. The hope is this will engage readers in personal reflection enabling them to consider their skills and attributes as leaders.

The roles and responsibilities of leaders include collaboratively working in teams, which is key to safe effective patient care. Different styles of leadership are adopted in different circumstances and it is important that leaders are aware of what style is being used and why in each situation.

Key Points

- In the rapidly changing horizon and demand of healthcare services, leadership is pivotal in providing a climate of psychological safety.
- Teamwork depends heavily on effective leadership.
- Every team member has leadership qualities and can lead when required.

References

Armstrong, A.E., 2007. Nursing Ethics: A Virtue-Based Approach. Palgrave Macmillan, Basingstoke.
Armstrong, A.E., 2006. Towards a strong virtue ethics for nursing practice. Nurs. Philos. 7 (3), 110–124.
Beauchamp, T.L., Childress, J.F., 2013. Principles of Biomedical Ethics, seventh ed. Oxford University Press, Oxford.
Bowie, P., 2010. Leadership and implementing a safety culture. Pract. Nurse 40 (10), 32–35.
Brafman, O., Beckstrom, R.A., 2006. The Starfish and the Spider: The Unstoppable Power of Leaderless Organizations. Penguin Books Ltd., London.
Bromiley, M., n.d. Independent report on the death of Elaine Bromiley. https://emcrit.org/wp-content/uploads/ElaineBromileyAnonymousReport.pdf (Accessed 30.10.23).
Brown, B., 2013. Daring Greatly. How the Courage to Be Vulnerable Transforms the Way We Live, Love, Parent and Lead. Penguin Books Ltd, London.
Brown, B., 2018. Dare to Lead. Brave work. Tough Conversations. Whole Hearts. Vermillion, London.
Burns, J.M., 1978. Leadership. Harper and Row, New York.
CIEHF, 2020. Rising to the challenge. Ergonomist 580, 6–7.
CIEHF, 2018. Human Factors for Health & Social Care White Paper. https://www.lboro.ac.uk/media/media/schoolanddepartments/design-and-creative-arts/downloads/CIEHF-2018-White-Paper_Human%20Factors-in-Health-Social-Care.pdf.
Civility Saves Lives Campaign. https://www.civilitysaveslives.com/.
Covey, S.R., 2020. The Seven Habits of Highly Effective People. Simon & Schuster, New York.
Dent, B., 2016. The power of a leadership philosophy. Nurse Lead 14 (6), 389–390.
Donaldson, L., 2002. An organisation with a memory. Clin. Med. 2 (5), 452–457.
Edmondson, A., 1999. Psychological Safety and Learning Behavior in Work Teams. Administrative Science Quarterly 44 (2), 350–383.

Edwards, S.D., 2009. Three versions of an ethics of care. Nurs. Philos 10 (4), 231–240.

Francis, R., 2013. Report of the Mid Staffordshire NHS Trust Public Inquiry-Executive Summary. The Stationery Office, London.

Goleman, D., 1998. Working with Emotional Intelligence. Bloomsbury Publishing, London.

Goss, S., 2015. Systems Leadership: A View from the Bridge. Office for Public Management, London.

Hammerly, M.E., Harmon, L., Schwaitzberg, S.D., 2014. Good to great: using 360-degree feedback to improve physician emotional intelligence. J. Healthc. Manag 59 (5), 354–366.

Heath, C., Heath, D., 2013. Decisive: How to Make Better Decisions and Choices in Life and Work. Crown Business, New York.

Heffernan, M., 2019. Wilful Blindness. Simon & Schuster, London.

Hignett, S., Edmonds, J., Herlihey, T., Pickup, L., Bye, R., Crumpton, E., et al., 2021. Human factors/ergonomics to support the design and testing of rapidly manufactured ventilators in the UK during the COVID-19 pandemic. Int. J. Qual. Health Care 12 (33 Suppl. 1), 4–10.

Lisle Baker, R., 2004. Using insights about perception and judgment from the Myers-Briggs Type Indicator Instrument as an aid to mediation. Harv. Negot. Law Rev 9, 115–186.

Luft, J., Ingham, H., 1955. The Johari window, a graphic model of interpersonal awareness. Proceedings of the Western Training Laboratory in Group Development. University of California, Los Angeles.

National Health Service Leadership Academy, 2024a. Talent Management Toolkit. https://www.leadershipacademy.nhs.uk/talent-management-hub/talent-management-toolkit-home-page/.

National Health Service Leadership Academy, 2024b. Healthcare Leadership Model. https://www.leadershipacademy.nhs.uk/healthcare-leadership-model/.

National Improvement and Leadership Development Board, 2016. Developing People – Improving Care. https://eoe.leadershipacademy.nhs.uk/wp-content/uploads/sites/6/2019/04/Developing_People-Improving_Care-010216.pdf.

Porath, C., 2016. Mastering Civility: A Manifesto for the Workplace. Grand Central Publishing, New York.

Reitz, M., Higgins, J., 2019. Speak up. Pearson Education Limited, Harlow.

Rogers, E., 1995. Diffusion of Innovations, fourth ed. The Free Press, New York.

Spears, L.C., 2010. Character and servant leadership: ten characteristics of effective, caring leaders. J. Virtue. Leadersh. 1, 25–30.

Syed, M., 2019. Rebel Ideas: The Power of Diverse Thinking. John Murray (Publishers), London.

Timms, M., 2016. Succession Planning that Works: The Critical Path of Leadership Development. Friesen-Press, Victoria.

Turner, C., n.d. When rudeness in teams turns deadly. https://www.ted.com/talks/chris_turner_when_rudeness_in_teams_turns_deadly?language=en (Accessed 30.10.23).

Trzeciak, S., Mazzarelli, A., 2019. Compassionomics: The Revolutionary Scientific Evidence that Caring Makes a Difference. Studer Group, Pensacola.

Weick, K.E., Sutcliffe, K.M., 2015. Managing the Unexpected: Sustained Performance in a Complex World, third ed. Wiley, Hoboken.

West, M., Eckert, R., Stewart, K., Pasmore, B., 2014. Developing collective leadership for healthcare. The King's Fund. Center for Creative Leadership. https://www.kingsfund.org.uk/sites/default/files/field/field_publication_file/developing-collective-leadership-kingsfund-may14.pdf.

West, M., 2020. Leading with compassion. Ergonomist 580, 12–13.

West, M.A., 2021. Compassionate Leadership. Sustaining Wisdom, Humanity and Presence in Health and Social Care. The Swirling Leaf Press.

Woodward, C., 2005. Winning!. Hodder & Stoughton, London.

CHAPTER 10

Culture in the Workplace

Margot Russell ■ Catie Paton

Introduction

Culture is a powerful element that can determine safety and quality of care in the workplace. Culture shapes teamwork and determines the types of professional relationship practitioners will adopt. West et al. (2020) describe culture in healthcare as being the determining factor for patient safety, and the importance of learning safety culture aspects in the workplace.

Resilience is a key human factors concept, which determines how individuals, teams and organisations monitor, adapt to and act on failures in stressful and high-risk situations. Resilience brings a new incentive to the table for focusing on continuous improvement rather than investigating practices when things go wrong. Resilience will benefit patient care and improve patient safety because the focus is on being proactive. Stress has been linked to patient safety outcomes, especially in high-risk environments concerning pressure, acuity of patient care and work volume. Recognising stress and fatigue in self, other individuals and the team as a nontechnical skill will be explored and coping mechanisms will be discussed in this chapter.

What Does Culture Mean?

When reports regarding concerns are published, one of the key areas for improvement cited is either organisational or workplace culture. The Francis Report regarding the failures in the Mid Staffordshire National Health Service (NHS) Trust, England (Department of Health, 2013), described numerous failings within the organisation, several of which discussed institutional culture placing business interests above that of patient care or staff well-being. The 2013 report of the Clostridium difficile outbreak and subsequent deaths at the Vale of Leven Hospital, Scotland, cites a culture wherein the hospital management and teams had lost their focus on delivering person-centred care and stopped listening to the concerns raised by staff and others (MacLean, 2014). The Okenden report published in 2022, following an inquiry into concerns regarding maternity services in Shrewsbury and Telford NHS Trust, England (Department of Health and Social Care, 2022), highlighted issues with the organisation's culture, and identified a 'them and us' culture being in place. These are some of the higher profile reports which highlight culture issues as significant contributing factors to the delivery of poor quality care and failures within the system. However, culture is something that is ill-defined and often better described when there are issues or challenges.

One of the reasons that culture is ill defined is because it means different things to different people. It is multifaceted and affected by people's own interpretations of what is happening. A number of different disciplines have attempted to define culture. The disciplines of anthropology, sociology and psychology have attempted to describe the components that contribute to culture; however, to date, there has been no consensus regarding its definition (Spencer-Oately, 2012).

EXERCISE 10.1

Discussion point: What does culture mean to you?

Consider the following and how they apply in healthcare settings:

Culture is made up of a set of attitudes, beliefs, values and behaviours shared by a group of people, interpreted by individuals and communicated to the next generation (Matsumoto,1996).

Culture is made up of three layers:

Visible manifestations: how things are organised, the way people dress, rituals and ceremonies.

Shared ways of thinking: the values and beliefs used to justify the visible manifestations and their associated behaviours such as views on autonomy and decisions of what needs to be done.

Deeper assumptions: what underpins daily life, such as role definitions and boundaries, expectations, knowledge and associated power in relationships (Mannion and Davies, 2018).

Being able to understand organisational cultures is essential to review and improve patient care and experience. It is also critical to understand how culture impacts the workplace and how we act and react within the health systems. Mannion and Davies's (2018) description of culture, which takes healthcare environments into consideration, can assist in giving us clues regarding organisational culture; this is presented in Table 10.1.

When thinking of the three components of culture, tools such as the '15 Steps Challenge' developed by NHS Health Education England (NHS HEE, 2017) provide a useful toolkit to start assessing environments and workplace culture. This tool, based on patient and caretaker feedback, works on the premise that patients and relatives make a determination about the quality of care and the experience they will have within 15 steps of walking into the clinical environment. To assist with its use, the tool is formatted into four sections.

The 15 Steps Challenge (Fig. 10.1) enables observers to examine the visible manifestations of the clinical environment culture. Observers are asked to notice signs such as what information is being displayed, are the clinical staff well-presented and how does the environment make them feel. In observing the interactions with patients, relatives and other staff members, observers are asked to consider the element of shared ways of thinking in the clinical culture. Prompts such as 'How are staff interacting with patients (are lower tones used for private conversations)?' and 'Are there any indicators that patients and carers are involved in their own care?' further assist assessing the workplace culture. The 15 Steps Challenge enables observers to clearly identify some of the deeper assumptions held within the workplace culture. Observers are asked to reflect on staff interactions to determine whether the teamwork is good and what types of behaviours are observed that may inspire confidence.

TABLE 10.1 ■ Description of Culture (Mannion and Davis, 2018)

Visible Manifestations	Shared Ways of Thinking	Deeper Assumptions
How does the environment look; is it organised? Is it clean?	Are there clear policies and standards that direct ways of working?	Are people clear about how each role in their part of the healthcare system contributes to the delivery of patient care and/or organisational priorities?
How does the environment feel; does it feel calm?	Are staff free to make informed decisions about priorities and care delivery?	Are professional boundaries clear and observable?
How do the staff look; are their uniforms clean and well-pressed? Are staff well-presented?	Are people involved in contributing to decisions, and share decision-making with people receiving care?	Is there flexibility to blur professional roles to ensure that safe, person-centred care is maintained?
Are people in certain roles identifiable, such as nurse, physiologist, doctor?	Are people involved and engaged in decisions about how the organisation can improve and shape priorities? If so, is it meaningful?	Is there a hierarchy evident in the system and does that assist or inhibit good communication and care?
How do people address each other? Are they friendly and professional or over familiar?	Are people clear about organisational priorities and able to articulate organisational values?	Does the environment promote continuous improvement in quality?
What other things do you notice about the care environment?		Does the environment promote continuous learning and development?

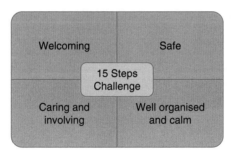

Fig. 10.1   15 Steps Challenge.

Such assessments tools enable appraisals of workplace cultures, although they are only useful if timely and constructive feedback is provided. The feedback assists the team to understand what has been observed and enables them to identify areas for learning and improvement.

Workplace Culture

Organisations should pay attention to clearly articulating their workplace culture. This means paying attention to the visual manifestations of the culture, understanding the shared ways of thinking and exploring the deeper assumptions identified in Fig. 10.2. Although we are focussing on healthcare organisations, it is relevant to organisations across all sectors.

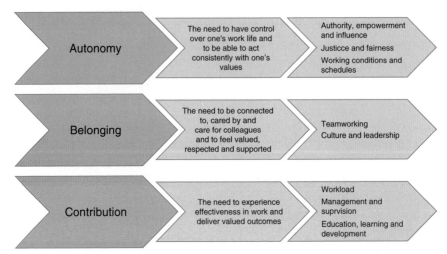

Fig. 10.2 Core needs of nurses and midwives. (West et al., 2020.)

'If you don't create the culture your staff will create one for you which might not be what you want'. Walt Disney

Disney is very clear in communicating their cultural identity and expectations at every opportunity and encourage their employees (or cast members) to ensure it is maintained at all levels of the organisation. In essence, they create an environment where their staff can address their core work needs.

When assessing workplace conditions, it is important to consider what the core needs at work should be. West et al. (2020) defined the core needs of nurses and midwives; however, it can be argued that those needs are not unique to these staff groups (Fig. 10.2).

Healthcare, by its very nature, relies on people interacting with one another—whether staff member to staff member, professional to professional, with patients, caretakers or family members. The way in which people experience those interactions is shaped by the context in which the interactions take place as well as the environment culture and organisation they take place in. Workplace conditions play a role in determining how effective these interactions are. Maben et al. (2023) suggest that how staff work together influences the ability of teams to be able to deliver safe, high quality care as well as their ability to learn from mistakes. They believe interactions are dependent on organisational factors such as leadership, clinical training and climate.

Therefore, how does this relate to the core needs at work? If we take a closer look at the key elements noted in the abovementioned framework and understand what the terms mean, we can better understand the connection of how this links to psychological safety and the human factors which impact workplace conditions.

Autonomy

Autonomy describes how people perceive their sphere of influence and levels of control in relation to ways of working, how care is delivered and how care is structured. If we perceive our sphere of influence as limited by the environment we work in, how likely are we to speak out when our values are under threat and we perhaps feel compromised?

EXERCISE 10.2

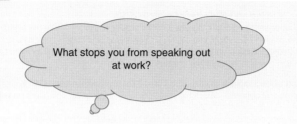

What stops you from speaking out at work?

In the codes of professional behaviour and ethics defined by healthcare regulators, there is a requirement for healthcare practitioners to raise and escalate concerns; however, reports—such as those mentioned earlier—have indicated that people find this difficult to implement (Table 10.2).

Despite professional obligations, there are other factors that impact the ability of an individual to speak out, which are revealed by asking questions such as:

- Do you feel psychologically safe to speak out?
- Do you fear repercussions if you speak out?
- Do other people not value what you seem to value, and do you feel you are not able to have any influence on what is going on?

All these factors are real considerations when we think about core needs at work. In a nutshell, we need to feel safe at work—both physically and psychologically.

Psychological Safety

The elements of autonomy, belonging and contribution all facilitate the creation of a psychologically safe working environment. Edmundson (2019) describes strategies that people use to survive in the workplace (Table 10.3).

This gives us insights into the second element of Mannion and Davies's (2018) definition of culture, 'shared ways of thinking'. What is done within local systems is as important as what is said. This also includes what is unsaid and what is implied, unconscious nuances, assumptions and expectations. Sometimes the drive for 'belonging' within a team impacts individual perceptions of psychological safety.

Belonging

Belonging describes the way in which teams work, their sense of purpose and how they consider the well-being of their members. How teams approach supporting well-being is key. Leadership that encourages a climate that enables team members to provide support and care to one another also notices the impact of delivering continuous improvements in the pursuit of high quality care.

However, one should not be misled into thinking that psychological safety is only about being 'nice' to people. In a psychologically safe environment, people are able to speak up and challenge one another in an attempt to learn from the different perspectives that individual team members contribute. There is a commonly held belief that not engaging in a certain way denies opportunities for learning and prevents opportunities to avoid 'preventable failures'. Psychologically safe teams regularly speak about errors and failures in an open and nonjudgemental way; the ethos is not to attribute blame but to understand the situation, its complexity and the interconnected contributory factors—the environmental and human factors at play.

TABLE 10.2 ■ The Code

Preserve safety: Nursing and Midwifery Council (2018)

You make sure that patient and public safety is not affected. You work within the limits of your competence, exercising your professional 'duty of candour' and raising concerns immediately whenever you come across situations that put patients or public safety at risk. You take necessary action to deal with any concerns where appropriate.

Report concerns about safety: Health and Care Professions Council (2016)

7.1 You must report any concerns about the safety or well-being of service users promptly and appropriately.

7.2 You must support and encourage others to report concerns and not prevent anyone from raising concerns.

7.3 You must take appropriate action if you have concerns about the safety or well-being of children or vulnerable adults.

7.4 You must make sure that the safety and well-being of service users always comes before any professional or other loyalties.

Follow up on such concerns

7.5 You must follow up on concerns that you have reported and, if necessary, escalate them.

7.6 You must acknowledge and act on concerns raised to you—investigating, escalating or dealing with those concerns where it is appropriate for you to do so.

Respond to risks to safety: General Medical Council (2020)

24 You must promote and encourage a culture that allows all staff to raise concerns openly and safely.

25 You must take prompt action if you think that patient safety, dignity or comfort is or may be seriously compromised.

TABLE 10.3 ■ Strategies to Survive in the Workplace (Edmundson, 2019)

Do Not Want to:	Do Not
Look ignorant	Ask questions
Look incompetent	Admit mistakes
Look disruptive	Make suggestions

EXERCISE 10.3

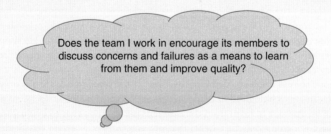

Does the team I work in encourage its members to discuss concerns and failures as a means to learn from them and improve quality?

The key to ensuring team that members feel like they belong is the leadership within the team. Leaders need to be role models and set the tone within the healthcare setting by encouraging and enabling discussions, constructive feedback and dialogue relating to identification of errors or near misses, early prevention of failures and areas for improving quality and experiences.

Edmundson (2019) has a toolkit that leaders and teams should consider (Table 10.4).

The tool kit assists in exposing the 'deeper assumptions' which inherently exist within the workplace culture. Whilst the onus is clearly placed on those in leadership roles to set the tone in the health and care environment, it is important that all members of the team engage in this approach and take individual responsibility for promoting the climate and culture within the team and organisation. If individuals are not in formal leadership positions, they can still contribute to creating a psychologically safe climate. The following list provides a good reminder of things teams and individual members can do:

- Ask questions
- Ensure you and others have a voice and that voice is heard
- Choose to listen actively and with curiosity
- Respond with interest and fascination
- Reframe the challenge to identify areas for learning and improvement
- Speak out
- Bring your true self to work (your values, beliefs and behaviours matter)

To ensure that a psychologically safe workplace is maintained, people and environments need to be resilient and offer meaningful contributions.

Contribution

For individuals to flourish at work, all the core work needs are required. Contribution describes the need to experience effectiveness in work and to be able to deliver valued outcomes—valued by the individual, team and organisation. A psychologically safe climate is imperative for achieving this; however, there are many other factors (Papadopoulou, 2023) that impact individual perceptions of meaningful contributions, one of which is resilience.

TABLE 10.4 ■ **Toolkit for Learning, Innovation and Growth (Edmundson, 2019)**

Setting the scene	Frame the work	Set expectations regarding failure and the need for continuous improvement
	Emphasise the purpose	Identify, with the team, what is at stake, why it matters and who it benefits
Inviting participants	Demonstrate situational humility	Acknowledge gaps and areas for improvement
	Practice inquiry	Ask questions with curiosity, practise active and intense listening
	Set up structures and processes	Create spaces and opportunities for staff to engage, provide guidelines and parameters for discussions
Respond productively	Express appreciation	Listen with intent, acknowledge contributions and show gratitude for participation
	Destigmatise failure	Look forward rather than continual reflection, offer help, discuss and identify next steps
	Sanction clear violations	Maintain consistent messaging about what is and is not acceptable

What Is Resilience?

Resilience is a prevalent term in healthcare environments, especially when situational pressures have intensified, particularly in the period just prior to as well as during the coronavirus disease 2019 (COVID-19) pandemic. We discuss personal resilience, developing resilience and resilience in the face of adversity; however, the focus tends to be on the individual.

Definitions of resilience tend to include the need for flexibility and adaptability, either from individuals or organisations, to cope with difficult or challenging experiences or periods of time and the ability to 'bounce back' (Weiss et al., 2023).

Taking the 'Safety II approach' into consideration and the definition offered by Hollnagel (2018), the study by Braithwaite et al. (2013) is a good starting point to understand resilience. They define resilience as the 'healthcare system's ability to adjust its functioning prior to, during, or following changes and disturbances, so that it can sustain required performance under both expected and unexpected conditions'. Resilience is not only about reducing risks and dangers; it should also encompass positive deviances and understanding successes so that 'work as imagined' and 'work as done' can be better aligned. Additionally, resilience engineering offers a system perspective wherein the whole organisation and system play roles rather than the frontline staff having the sole responsibility. To perform resiliently at all levels, Hollnagel (2018) proposes that organisations must:

- Anticipate: prepare for the unexpected, simulate it and learn to work through issues prior to real life events
- Monitor: collect meaningful data so that we know where we are and what to look for so that we can respond
- Respond: able to adjust to eventualities and disturbances when they happen
- Learning: lessons from positive and negative experiences must be translated to training, policies and guidelines

Resilience engineering can be specifically applied to improve quality and safety of care such as the CARE (Concepts for Applying Resilience Engineering) model (Anderson et al., 2016). This model assists in increasing resilience in practice through mechanisms such as aligning mismatches between demand and capacity.

Whilst there are also other definitions of resilience, the words in Fig. 10.3 are often used to describe what is meant by or related to the term.

An example of the concept individual resilience is linked closely to various workplace conditions.

All three factors identified in Fig. 10.4 can positively or negatively impact perceptions of well-being and resilience, and can influence how well individual healthcare practitioners cope in challenging circumstances. The impact of high levels of job demands can often be cushioned by some of the job resources available within an organisation. Access to peer support networks and supportive structures such as clinical or professional supervision can assist in rebalancing the negative impacts of high demand jobs. However, it is recognised that during such times of high pressure and high work demand, organisations and staff are unlikely to make time to undertake supportive mechanisms, such as supervision, and facilitate peer support networks. Subsequently, this can lead to an increase in stress and poor staff well-being (Martin and Snowden, 2020).

It is essential that time for supervision is valued and prioritised within organisations as a means of ensuring and maintaining physical and psychological safety when there are periods of high demand or pressure.

To balance the demands of a job, besides offering resources to ensure supportive mechanisms and infrastructure to support staff, it is essential to connect purpose and meaning to the work to be done; the organisation's values, along with the individuals' sense of purpose, enable individuals to connect with their own sense of purpose and motivation to work within healthcare.

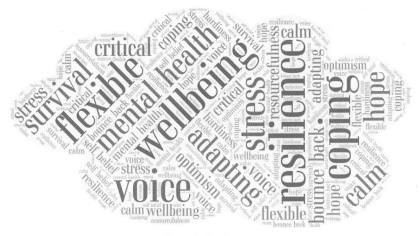

Fig. 10.3 Resilience.

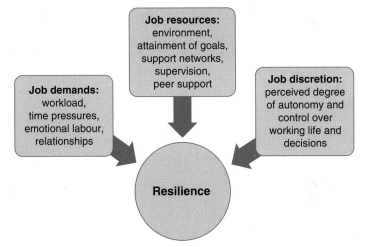

Fig. 10.4 Factors that impact individual resilience.

EXERCISE 10.4

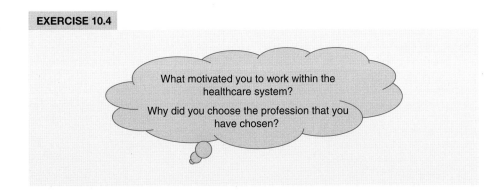

The final element to consider that impacts resilience is the extent of control that individuals perceive they have in decision-making and over their working lives. Workplace cultures which limit the ability of individuals to retain a degree of self-direction and autonomy for prolong periods of time lead to decreased levels of job satisfaction and poor perceptions of self-worth (Gottlieb et al., 2022). This was very much apparent during the COVID-19 pandemic when healthcare systems moved into command-and-control structures in an attempt to react and respond to the uncertainties of the situation. Decisions were often made at pace, without consultation and with limited information or with information that changed frequently, such as guidance regarding management of the care environment. Staff reported high levels of burnout and fatigue as the pandemic progressed. Healthcare staff at all levels experienced a decreased ability to control the work they were required to undertake or their workplace environment, and as a result their resilience was impacted significantly.

Whilst autonomy plays a major role in determining workplace culture, healthcare relies on an interdependence between and across professional staff groups. Gittell (2016) recognises the importance of autonomy in supporting resilience within healthcare settings, but argues that the need to maintain relationships has a greater impact when supporting a more resilient workplace culture.

Heffernan (2015) describes the benefits for organisations that invest in the social connections of their workforce. She highlights the benefits of building trust, a sense of shared values and a culture of reciprocity in supporting both individual and organisational resilience. Heffernan argues that without such investment, a climate of safety will not flourish. Furthermore, she describes the need to develop and foster a sense of togetherness and take time for 'collective restoration'. In doing so, the workplace culture moves from being task- and transaction-orientated to relationship-focussed. This is essential within healthcare if we are to reduce risks and improve safety.

Joy in Work

It may seem an odd choice of phrase and not one commonly expressed or associated to work; however, joy in work is key to supporting and promoting safe, effective and person-centred caring working cultures—caring for practitioners as well as caring for patients. It encompasses the human factors and nontechnical skills required to create environments that thrive rather than just survive.

In 2017, the Institute for Healthcare Improvement (IHI) (Perlo et al., 2017) published a white paper describing a framework for improving joy in work. IHI recognised the challenge of burnout in healthcare professionals and the subsequent impact on safe and reliable person-centred care delivery. Table 10.5 presents how burnout can impact patient care.

IHI recognised the scale of the challenge that existed and chose to reframe attention from focussing on ways to address staff burnout to reconnecting people to the purpose and meaning within their roles. Reframing the conversation to contemplate joy encouraged practitioners, managers and wider healthcare systems to consider positive approaches towards improvement.

EXERCISE 10.5

'Joy is more than the absence of burnout'.
IHI (2017)

Reflect on this question for a couple of moments:
What does joy in work mean to you?

TABLE 10.5 ■ **Some Impacts of Burnout**

Impact on Healthcare Practitioners	Impact on Colleagues	Impact on Patient Care
Physical exhaustion	Increased absenteeism or presenteeism, thus increasing work pressures for others	Lapses in concentration causing errors
Insomnia	Lack of civility experienced	Lack of empathy
Headaches	Decreased sense of psychological safety	Depersonalising the individual
Decreasing mental health	Unwillingness to speak out	Poor experience of care
Substance misuse	Less sense of team	Poor patient outcomes
Reduced commitment to work	Poor social connectedness	Less informed regarding care
Inability to concentrate	Fragmentation of team working	Decrease in satisfaction
Poor job satisfaction		Increase in complaints

IHI recognised the need to provide a framework and support to assist people to understand the concepts. When examining the framework, it is clear IHI is encouraging organisations and practitioners to consider the workplace culture within which they provide patient care.

Fig. 10.5 presents the framework that provides those in leadership positions with some clarity regarding the key elements which they should focus on. It identifies the main components that contribute to making a workplace culture effective and safe for patients and staff alike and joyful to work within.

The framework highlights the nine key elements that IHI believes contribute to creating safe, effective and person-centred environments; they are very clear in articulating the role of the leader in creating and maintaining the conditions for joy in work to flourish.

West (2021) encourages leaders to work at all levels across the organisation and practice compassionate leadership as a means to support and drive safe care environments—safe for staff as well as patients. Table 10.6 presents as model by West (2021) that assists leaders (and others) to promote and support safe person-centred care environments.

These four elements by West (2021) mirror the four pillars that IHI suggests leaders to implement when embedding joy in work:

- Ask staff, 'What matters to you?' 'What makes a good day for you?' 'When we are at our best?' 'What does this look like?'
- Identify local impediments to joy in work: What are the pebbles (or boulders) in your shoes?
- Commit to shared responsibility at all levels in the organisation; ensure staff engagement and shared decision-making in promoting joy in work.
- Use improvement science to test approaches and impact; real time measures, tracked over time.

Why Is This Important?

Considering the definition of culture by Mannion and Davies (2018), it is clear that the components that contribute to the creation of workplace cultures also greatly impact human factors. It is essential to pay attention to the signals within a workplace that begin to articulate what is valued and what is being valued by the organisation and people who work within it. This can range from how the physical environment looks, smells and feels to how people interact with one another and the evident relationships.

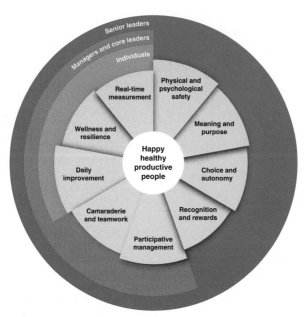

Fig. 10.5 Framework for happy, healthy and productive people. (Perlo et al., 2017.)

TABLE 10.6 ■ **Four Elements of Compassionate Leadership (West, 2021)**

Activity	Behaviours
Attending	Paying attention to the situation and the pressures staff are experiencing: workload, stress, staffing issues, symptoms of burnout
	Listening with fascination
	Listening without judgement to what is said and what is left unsaid
Understanding	Engaging and supportive leadership
	Enabling and creating a climate for staff to feel and be empowered
	Teaching approaches used to assist staff in identifying solutions for themselves
	Recognising the benefits of working collectively to seek solutions
Empathising	Viewing the situation from another perspective by being present in their 'world'
	Supporting and promoting trust and psychological safety
	Practising social connectedness and positive relationships
	Making staff feel valued, respected and engaged in the team
Helping	Taking intelligent and meaningful action to help
	Removing obstacles and barriers that detract from the 'real work' of the team
	Assisting staff to critically evaluate options and solutions rather than imposing a way forward

When systems are under extreme pressure, as has been the case during the COVID-19 pandemic, sense of autonomy, belonging and contribution of individuals are significantly impacted. This further impacts individual resilience and, if prolonged, organisational resilience.

It is well recognised that stress and work pressures significantly reduce individual situational awareness—the ability to understand the world around and make sense of the working environment. This can lead to lapses in concentration, fatigue, reduced awareness of time and subsequently catastrophic failures in patient care if it is not addressed (Kelly et al., 2023).

Tools and frameworks such as the 15 Steps Challenge and those by IHI assist in maintaining focus on workplace culture and early intervention to prevent harm to staff and patients. However, attention to culture and environmental factors must be constant. West (2021) argues that compassionate leadership is not just the domain of those in formal or hierarchical leadership positions, but is a shared responsibility for all members of staff.

To ensure that compassionate cultures are supported and maintained, the need for people to focus on relationships and relational care is necessary. Healthcare delivery that is based on shared values, trust and respect is recognised as decreasing harm, enhancing safety and improving patient outcomes. Within these workplaces, it is important that people recognise when colleagues need help and support and take action to provide compassionate leadership at an individual level.

Clinical supervision and peer support networks provide mechanisms to enable discussions regarding stress and resilience to take place and are essential to ensuring safety. There are other tools which may assist individuals in creating space and focus on maintaining a sense of purpose and autonomy in their work—thereby reducing stress and burnout.

West (2021) highlights the need for 'self-compassion', recognising that as individuals we are flawed, vulnerable and prone to failure. Furthermore, he suggests that being aware of the impact our behaviours have on ourselves and others brings an honesty and authenticity to the workplace, and consequently impacts the culture within which we work. Practicing mindfulness or values-based reflective practice assist us in identifying and connecting with ourselves, increasing our awareness and understanding our reactions and feelings, especially in pressured and stressful situations.

Exploring Self Compassion: RAIN
(West, 2021)

Take some time to pause and reflect on the following:

R – recognising what is happening for me in this moment; be aware and present with your feelings

A – allowing or accepting what is happening without judgement

I – investigating or inquiring into emotions and feelings; being curious about what they represent and how they feel

N – nurture self-compassion; nurturing of self in context of feelings, self-soothing statements that encourage the best in ourselves by being present

---

Recognising when colleagues are under pressure and supporting one another further assists in the building of a safety culture within organisations—psychologically and physically. Simple tools such as the 'Going Home Checklist' help individuals to recognise the feelings they experience, develop awareness of colleagues and encourage checking in with them before going home at the end of the shift or day (Doncaster and Bassetlaw Teaching Hospitals NHS Foundation Trust, 2019).

Conclusion

It is essential to understand what is meant when discussing workplace culture. The signs and symbols of workplace cultures are ever present and easily identifiable from the aesthetics of messages and environment to the way relationships are portrayed and displayed and the language used. These signs and symbols give observers insights into what and whose voice is being valued in an environment.

Culture is not a static entity; it is impacted by individual perceptions of autonomy, belonging and contribution to the workplace. Consequently, workplace culture influences both systems and personal resilience, which subsequently have a direct impact on the delivery of safe and person-centred care and the psychological safety of those that provide it.

By using the frameworks such as IHI's 'joy in work', workplace culture can be improved; such improvements can be measured to identify the impact on individuals, teams and the wider healthcare system. Furthermore, these improvements impact perceptions of stress and fatigue. Promoting activities such as mindfulness, values-based reflective practice and self-compassion can assist practitioners in improving their situational awareness—thus further enhancing patient safety.

Key Points

- Culture is important in ensuring staff and patient safety
- Culture can be assessed and reviewed
- Culture can be improved by systems approaches as well individual activities which enhance resilience and well-being

References

Anderson, J.E., Ross, A.J., Back, J., Duncan, M., Snell, P., Walsh, K., et al., 2016. Implementing resilience engineering for healthcare quality improvement using the CARE model: a feasibility study protocol. Pilot. Feasibility. Stud. 2 (1), 61.

Braithwaite, J., Wears, R.L., Hollnagel, E., 2013. Resilient Health Care. Ashgate Publishing Group, Farnham.

Department of Health, 2013. Report of the Mid Staffordshire NHS Foundation Trust Public Inquiry February 2013 Executive Summary. The Stationery Office, London. https://assets.publishing.service.gov.uk/government/uploads/system/uploads/attachment_data/file/279124/0947.pdf.

Department of Health and Social Care, 2022. The Final Report of the Ockenden Review: Findings, Conclusions and Essential Actions from the Independent Review of Maternity Services at the Shrewsbury and Telford Hospital NHS Trust. https://www.gov.uk/government/publications/final-report-of-the-ockenden-review.

Doncaster and Bassetlaw Teaching Hospitals NHS Foundation Trust, 2019. Going home Checklist. https://www.dbth.nhs.uk/news/the-going-home-checklist/.

Edmundson, A.C., 2019. The Fearless Organisation. Creating Psychological Safety in the Workplace for Learning, Innovation and Growth. John Wiley & Sons, New Jersey.

General Medical Council, 2020. Good Medical Practice. https://www.gmc-uk.org/-/media/documents/good-medical-practice---english-20200128_pdf-51527435.pdf.

Gittell, J.H., 2016. Rethinking autonomy: relationships as a source of resilience in a changing healthcare system. Health Serv. Res. 51 (5), 1701–1705.

Gottlieb, L.N., Gottlieb, B., Bitzas, V., 2022. Creating empowering conditions for nurses with workplace autonomy and agency: how healthcare leaders could be guided by Strengths-Based Nursing and Healthcare Leadership (SBNH-L). J. Healthc. Leadersh. 13, 169–181.

Health and Care Professions Council, 2016. Standards of Conduct, Performance and Ethics. https://www.hcpc-uk.org/globalassets/resources/standards/standards-of-conduct-performance-and-ethics.pdf.

Heffernan, M., 2015. Beyond Measure: The Big Impact of Small Changes. Simon & Schuster, London.

Hollnagel, E., 2018. Safety-II in Practice: Developing the Resilience Potentials. Routledge, London.

Kelly, F.E., Frerk, C., Bailey, C.R., Cook, T.M., Ferguson, K., Flin, R., et al., 2023. Human factors in anaesthesia: a narrative review. Anaesthesia 78 (4), 479–490.

Maben, J., Ball, J., Edmundson, A., 2023. Elements of Improving Quality and Safety in Healthcare: Workplace Conditions. Cambridge University Press, Cambridge.

MacLean, R.N.M., 2014. The Vale of Leven Hospital Inquiry Report. https://hub.careinspectorate.com/media/1415/vale-of-leven-hospital-inquiry-report.pdf.

Mannion, R., Davies, H., 2018. Understanding organisational culture for healthcare quality improvement. BMJ. 363, k4907.

Martin, P., Snowdon, D., 2020. Can clinical supervision bolster clinical skills and well-being through challenging times? J. Adv. Nurs. 76 (11), 2781–2782.

Matsumoto, D., 1996. Culture and Psychology. Brooks/Cole, Pacific Grove.

National Health Service England, 2017. The 15 Steps challenge: Quality from a Patient's Perspective; an Inpatient Toolkit. https://www.england.nhs.uk/wp-content/uploads/2017/11/15-steps-inpatient.pdf.

Nursing and Midwifery Council (NMC), 2018. Read the Code Online. https://www.nmc.org.uk/standards/code/read-the-code-online/.

Papadopoulou, A., 2023. The Relationship between Work Engagement and Meaningful Work to Well-Being and Aspiration Index in the Health Field: The Case of Physicians. Research Square (preprint) https://www.researchgate.net/publication/367060110_The_Relationship_Between_Work_Engagement_and_Meaninful_Work_to_Well-Being_and_Aspiration_Index_in_the_Health_Field_The_Case_of_Psycisians.

Perlo, J., Balik, B., Swenson, S., Kabcenell, A., Landsman, J., Feely, D., 2017. IHI Framework for Improving Joy in Work. IHI White Paper. Institute for Healthcare Improvement, Cambridge, Massachusetts.

Spencer-Oatey, H., 2012. What Is Culture? A Compilation of Quotations. GlobalPAD Core Concepts. https://warwick.ac.uk/fac/soc/al/globalpad-rip/openhouse/interculturalskills_old/core_concept_compilations/global_pad_-_what_is_culture.pdf.

Weiss, S.S., Weiss, L., Clayton, R., Ruble, M.J., Cole, J.D., 2023. The relationship between pharmacist resilience, burnout, and job performance. J. Pharm. Pract. [published online ahead of print, 20 Mar 2023], 8971900231164886.

West, M., Bailey, S., Williams, E., 2020. The Courage of Compassion: Supporting Nurses and Midwives to Deliver High Quality Care. The King's Fund. https://. www.kingsfund.org.uk/sites/default/files/2020-09/The%20courage%20of%20compassion%20full%20report_0.pdf.

West, M.A., 2021. Compassionate Leadership: Sustaining Wisdom, Humanity and Presence in Health and Social Care. Swirling Leaf Press.

Going home checklist

✓ Take a moment to think about today.

✓ Acknowledge one thing that was difficult during your working day - let it go.

✓ Consider three things that went well.

✓ Check on your colleagues before you leave - are they OK?

✓ Are you OK? Your senior team are here to support you.

✓ Now switch your attention to home - rest and recharge.

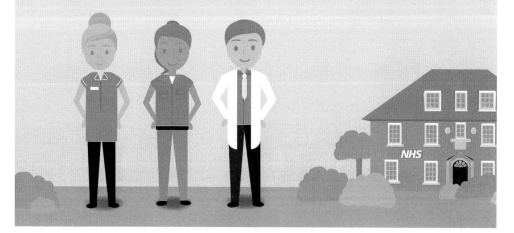

Page numbers followed by "*b*" indicate boxes, "*f*" indicate figures, "*t*" indicate tables.